TEXTBOOK OF
BASIC NURSING

Seventh Edition

Joyce Young Johnson, Ph.D, RN
Adjunct Faculty
School of Nursing
Georgia State University
Atlanta, Georgia

Resource Nurse
Nursing Service
Crawford Long Hospital of Emory University

Phyllis Prather Hicks, RN, BSN
Nursing Instructor
Harrisburg Community College
Harrisburg, Pennsylvania

Visit the Lippincott's NursingCenter Website
http://www.nursingcenter.com

Visit the Lippincott Williams and Wilkins Website
http://www.lww.com

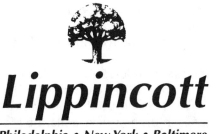

Lippincott

Philadelphia • New York • Baltimore

Ancillary Editor: Doris S. Wray
Project Editor: Nicole Walz
Senior Production Manager: Helen Ewan
Production Coordinator: Nannette Winski
Design Coordinator: Doug Smock
Compositor: Pine Tree Composition, Inc.
Printer/Binder: Victor Graphics, Inc.

7th Edition

9 8 7 6 5 4 3 2 1

ISBN 0-781-71857-0

Care has been taken to confirm the accuracy of the information presented
and to describe generally accepted practices. However, the authors, editors,
and publisher are not responsible for errors or omissions or for any consequences from application of the information in this book and make no war-
ranty, express or implied, with respect to the contents of the publication.

The authors, editors and publisher have exerted every effort to ensure that
drug selection and dosage set forth in this text are in accordance with current recommendations and practice at the time of publication. However, in
view of ongoing research, changes in government regulations, and the constant flow of information relating to drug therapy and drug reactions, the
reader is urged to check the package insert for each drug for any changes in
indications and dosage and for added warnings and precautions. This is particularly important when the recommended agent is a new or infrequently
employed drug.

Some drugs and medical devices presented in this publication have Food
and Drug Administration (FDA) clearance for limited use in restricted research settings. It is the responsibility of the health care provider to ascertain
the FDA status of each drug or device planned for use in their clinical practice.

Praises and glory to God the Father, Son, and Holy Spirit who guide and direct my life. Thank you to my husband, Larry, and my children, Virginia and Larry Jr., for your love—you are my greatest joy. To my parents, Dorothy and Riley Young Sr., my sisters and brother, family, and friends, thank you for your love and support.

JOYCE

Thank you to my husband, Rick, for his encouragement, support, patience, and extraordinary PC skills. To my children, Felicia, Stephanie, Georgi, and Gabriel: Thank you for all the hugs, kisses, and extra time on the computer you gave me! To my friends in the Nursing Department of Harrisburg Area Community College who have always encouraged, uplifted, and supported me. A special thank you to my parents, James and Georgia Prather who taught me to love God, work hard, and believe in myself.

PHYLLIS

To the students, we wish you a wonderful educational experience and a glorious career in nursing. We hope you enjoy using your Study Guide.

JOYCE AND PHYLLIS

Acknowledgments

Many thanks to Doris Wray for her direction and support throughout this endeavor—your energy is inspiring!

Thanks to Clemmie Riggins and Rick Hicks for their computer expertise and wonderful clerical assistance!

Contents

UNIT XIII: Assisting the Older Person

UNIT XIV: Mental Health

UNIT XV: The Client in a Variety of Settings

Part D PERSONAL RESPONSIBILITIES OF THE GRADUATE NURSE

UNIT XVI: The Transition From Student to Graduate Nurse

Introduction

This study guide is designed to help the student master the content in the text-book and is based on principles used in nursing education. The student will use these general concepts and incorporate them with practice exercises based on content from Carolyn Bunker Rosdahl's *Textbook of Basic Nursing,* seventh edition. The study guide authors used basic concepts relevant to learning and applying nursing knowledge to select or to create activities and projects that will help the student study effectively. Emphasis is also given to test taking skills that will help the student demonstrate understanding of the content on exams.

An important part of learning in nursing education is directed toward improving reading and vocabulary skills. Students who focus on the following KEY areas when studying will find it easier to manage the large amount of new vocabulary and the many new ideas they must assimilate. Thus, this study guide is divided into three parts.

Section One provides basic exercises and guidance on how to study effectively. The exercises in Section One should be used to help the student develop reading and study skills and to prepare for Section Two.

In *Section Two,* practice exercises are provided for each chapter and are structured according to key learning concepts and skills. Section Two is organized around the following important study skills:

Improving Concentration

Vocabulary Development

Reading Comprehension

Study Skills

Test-Taking Strategies

Section Two contains study guide activities for each chapter of the textbook. Each chapter contains a variety of drills and activities based on the first three areas in the list above. All exercises in the study guide also demonstrate some or a combination of the above areas. The questions posed in the study guide, for example, will help to prepare the student to respond to different types of quizzes or tests he or she might have in a course or nursing program.

Section Three expands on content in Chapter 99, Career Opportunities and Job Seeking, of the textbook. Exercises and samples of job postings, cover letters, resumés and other job search related materials are provided.

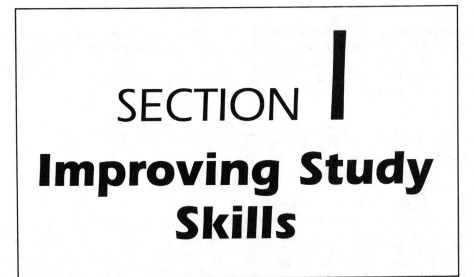

SECTION I
Improving Study Skills

IMPROVING CONCENTRATION

Improving your concentration while studying helps you study most efficiently. Improving concentration involves planning for regular study periods, choosing a location which will help you study, and developing good habits that help you read and understand more effectively.

- Analyze your own study habits. Are you a morning or an evening person? Schedule your study periods when you will be most alert.
- Plan your study periods. Be realistic about the amount of time it takes to read and review a chapter. If you have not developed the habit of keeping a written schedule or agenda, now is a good time to do so. Writing down your personal and academic appointments in one central place will help to keep you organized. If you are a busy family member with responsibilities to children, spouse, or other family members, establish a family calendar that shows everyone when you have scheduled your study periods.
- Create a place to study. If you have a room in which you can set up a desk or table that is just for studying and have a bookcase in which you keep all your textbooks, class handouts, notes, and other materials, great. You may, however, need to create a study area on the dining room or kitchen table, or you may find that the library is the only quiet place that you have available. The important principle is to have a time and place that means study to you, in which you will not be interrupted by family, television, or other temptations.

READING PREPARATION EXERCISE

Each chapter in your textbook begins with Keys For Learning and includes several features to help you understand the chapters. Before reading a chapter, spend 10 minutes (check your clock or set a timer) gaining an overview of what the chapter is about. Scan the chapter, reading the Objectives, Key Terms, Topic Outline, and the major headings and subheadings in the chapter. Scan the Key Points at the end of the chapter.

This overview will help focus your concentration on the areas you are about to read.

USING THE STUDY GUIDE

The first exercise for each chapter deals with beginning to understand major content and key points. These exercises will help you become more focused and organized in studying and help you be an active, rather than a passive, reader. Use the first exercises in each study guide chapter to prepare for studying the entire chapter.

Vocabulary Development

The second section of each study guide chapter focuses on vocabulary development to help you learn and remember the specialized vocabulary used in nursing, medicine, and health care settings. Each chapter in the textbook begins with a list of Key Terms and within the chapter these are first highlighted in **boldface type.** Each term is also defined in the Glossary at the end of your textbook. The study guide exercises vary from identifying words from definitions, solving word scrambles, matching, to other creative activities.

Each chapter in the study guide includes a list of abbreviations and acronyms with definitions used in that chapter. To check your knowledge, cover the definitions and see if you can identify what each abbreviation or acronym means.

The following exercise is suggested for every chapter you read:

While reading and highlighting your text (highlighting is discussed below), note the presence of the Key Terms. Underline these with a red fine tip marker. Also underline the descriptive words. For example:

Hippocratic oath—underline the words *physician, principles, enter field of medicine* (Chapter 1, page 3)

Holistic health care—*caring for the whole person* (Chapter 1, page 4)

Reading Comprehension

Reading comprehension is improved, first by knowing the vocabulary and, second, by *reading actively*. Active reading means thinking about what you are reading and asking yourself questions to be sure you are understanding what you read.

To help focus and improve comprehension, practice the following techniques:

Highlighting. Use a multi-color pack of high-lighters. Proper use of highlighting technique will train your eyes to note the most important information contained on each page. To remind you to high-light, you will see an icon at some point in each study guide chapter.

1. Choose one color highlighter and highlight the most important words in the learning objectives. For example, in Chapter One in the textbook, Objective 2 is:

"Describe Florence Nightingale's influence on mod-ern nursing practice."

What are the most important words to highlight in the Objective?

Nightingale's, influence, nursing practice

2. Using the same color, highlight content in the chapter related to the objective. Remember that you **always** read the text one time through first, to deter-mine the most important words, phrases, or terms. Then, read the text, highlighting the most important ideas.

Remember to highlight main points in short bursts, highlighting only essential words and phrases. High-lighting entire sentences or paragraphs defeats the purpose! The correct use of highlighting is helpful when you review material you have studied earlier—the important points are already marked for you.

Highlighting Exercise

Remember that you always read the text one time through first to determine the most important words, phrases or terms. Then, read the text again, highlighting the most important ideas. Then, read the following text, highlighting the most important terms and/or ideas. Then reread and highlight more, if necessary. Then, compare with the sample on the back of this page to see if you agree about the most important ideas.

Florence Nightingale

Even during the days when nursing was considered menial and undesirable, some women continued to care for the sick. Probably the most famous was Florence Nightingale (Fig. 1-1). Most nurses before her time received almost no training. Not until she graduated from Kaiserswerth and began to teach her concepts did nursing become a respected profession.

Nightingale was born in Italy in 1820 to wealthy English parents. When she was still very young, her parents returned to England. In 1844, an American doctor visited the family, and Nightingale asked him if entering the field of nursing would be appropriate for her. The reply from Dr. Samuel Gridley Howe has become a classic quotation. He said:

> My dear Miss Florence, it would be unusual (for you to enter nursing), and in England whatever is unusual is apt to be thought unsuitable; but I say to you, go forward, if you have a vocation for that way of life; act up to your aspiration and you will find that there is never anything unbecoming or unladylike in doing your duty for the good of others. Choose your path, go on with it, wherever it may lead you, and God be with you!

In 1851, Nightingale entered the Deaconess School in Kaiserswerth. She was 31 years old, and her family and friends were strongly opposed to her becoming a nurse. After her graduation in 1853, she became superintendent of a charity hospital for governesses. She trained her attendants on the job and greatly improved the quality of care. In 1854, the Crimean War began. During this conflict Nightingale gained fame. She entered the battlefield near Scutari, Turkey with 38 other nurses and cared for the sick and injured. The nurses had few supplies and little outside support. Nonetheless, Nightingale insisted on establishing sanitary conditions and providing good nursing care, which immediately reduced the mortality rate. Her persistence made her famous and she and her nurses were greatly admired. Her dedicated service both during the day and at night, when she and her nurses made their rounds carrying oil lamps, created a public image of "the lady with the lamp." In time the "Nightingale lamp" became the symbol of nursing. Today, many schools of nursing display a model of the lamp or a picture of Florence Nightingale carrying a lamp.

Nightingale's Definition of Nursing

Nightingale had definite and progressive ideas about nursing. Her definition of nursing, published in 1859, is still important today. She said, "Nature alone cures. Surgery removes the bullet out of the limb, which is an obstruction to cure, but nature heals the wounds . . . . Medicine assists nature to remove the obstruction, but does nothing more. And what nursing has to do in either case, is to put the patient in the best condition for nature to act upon him" (Nightingale, 1992, pp. 74–75).

The Nightingale School

Building on the respect she had established in the Crimean War, Nightingale opened the first nursing school outside a hospital in 1860. The nursing course was 1 year in length and included both classroom and clinical experience, a major innovation at that time. Students gained clinical experience at St. Thomas Hospital in London. Because it was financially independent, the school emphasized learning, rather than service to the hospital. Some principles of the Nightingale School for Nurses are still taught today. Examples include:

- Cleanliness is vital to recovery.
- The sick person is an individual with individual needs.
- Nursing is an art and a science.
- Nurses should spend their time caring for others, not cleaning.
- Prevention is better than cure.
- The nurse must work as a member of a team.
- The nurse must use discretion, but must follow the physician's orders.
- Self-discipline and self-evaluation are important.
- A good nursing program encourages a nurse's individual development.
- The nurse should be healthy in mind and body.
- Teaching is part of nursing.
- Nursing is a specialty.
- A nurse does not "graduate," but continues to learn throughout his or her career. Nursing curricula should include both theoretical knowledge and practical experience.

3. Choose a different color highlighter for each objective and move through the learning objectives. By the time you finish the chapter, you will know that you have covered all the objectives for the chapter.

4. Complete all the exercises for a chapter in the Study Guide, without looking up any answers. If you are not required to turn them in as assignments, you might use a study buddy or a study group to check your Study Guide exercises. Exchange papers in the group and discuss your answers. A study buddy or study group can be challenging and fun.

Florence Nightingale

Even during the days when nursing was considered menial and undesirable, some women continued to care for the sick. Probably the most famous was Florence Nightingale (Fig. 1-1). Most nurses before her time received almost no training. Not until she graduated from Kaiserswerth and began to teach her concepts did nursing become a respected profession.

Nightingale was born in Italy in 1820 to wealthy English parents. When she was still very young, her parents returned to England. In 1844, an American doctor visited the family, and Nightingale asked him if entering the field of nursing would be appropriate for her. The reply from Dr. Samuel Gridley Howe has become a classic quotation. He said:

> My dear Miss Florence, it would be unusual (for you to enter nursing), and in England whatever is unusual is apt to be thought unsuitable; but I say to you, go forward, if you have a vocation for that way of life; act up to your aspiration and you will find that there is never anything unbecoming or unladylike in doing your duty for the good of others. Choose your path, go on with it, wherever it may lead you, and God be with you!

In 1851, Nightingale entered the Deaconess School in Kaiserswerth. She was 31 years old, and her family and friends were strongly opposed to her becoming a nurse. After her graduation in 1853, she became superintendent of a charity hospital for governesses. She trained her attendants on the job and greatly improved the quality of care. In 1854, the Crimean War began. During this conflict Nightingale gained fame. She entered the battlefield near Scutari, Turkey with 38 other nurses and cared for the sick and injured. The nurses had few supplies and little outside support. Nonetheless, Nightingale insisted on establishing sanitary conditions and providing good nursing care, which immediately reduced the mortality rate. Her persistence made her famous and she and her nurses were greatly admired. Her dedicated service both during the day and at night, when she and her nurses made their rounds carrying oil lamps, created a public image of "the lady with the lamp." In time the "Nightingale lamp" became the symbol of nursing. Today, many schools of nursing display a model of the lamp or a picture of Florence Nightingale carrying a lamp.

Nightingale's Definition of Nursing

Nightingale had definite and progressive ideas about nursing. Her definition of nursing, published in 1859, is still important today. She said, "Nature alone cures. Surgery removes the bullet out of the limb, which is an obstruction to cure, but nature heals the wounds . . . . Medicine assists nature to remove the obstruction, but does nothing more. And what nursing has to do in either case, is to put the patient in the best condition for nature to act upon him" (Nightingale, 1992, pp. 74–75).

The Nightingale School

Building on the respect she had established in the Crimean War, Nightingale opened the first nursing school outside a hospital in 1860. The nursing course was 1 year in length and included both classroom and clinical experience, a major innovation at that time. Students gained clinical experience at St. Thomas Hospital in London. Because it was financially independent, the school emphasized learning, rather than service to the hospital. Some principles of the Nightingale School for Nurses are still taught today. Examples include:

- Cleanliness is vital to recovery.
- The sick person is an individual with individual needs.
- Nursing is an art and a science.
- Nurses should spend their time caring for others, not cleaning.
- Prevention is better than cure.
- The nurse must work as a member of a team.
- The nurse must use discretion, but must follow the physician's orders.
- Self-discipline and self-evaluation are important.
- A good nursing program encourages a nurse's individual development.
- The nurse should be healthy in mind and body.
- Teaching is part of nursing.
- Nursing is a specialty.
- A nurse does not "graduate," but continues to learn throughout his or her career. Nursing curricula should include both theoretical knowledge and practical experience.

STUDY SKILLS

Taking care of yourself can make the most effective use of your study time. The basics of keeping healthy apply to nursing students, too! Refer to Chapter 6—Health and Wellness in your textbook and plan ways you will promote and protect your own health.

Two special notations:

1. Avoid excessive snacks.
2. If you smoke, quit. If you have recently quit, keep it that way.

Studying can become very stressful, especially for students who are juggling family and employment responsibilities. Excess snacking and smoking are short-term stress relief mechanisms, but can cause long-term damage to your energy and health. You may think that quitting smoking and entering your practical/vocational nursing program would be too much stress at one time. However, nearly all nursing schools, hospitals, and other health care settings do not allow smoking and you may find that the required periods without smoking can help you quit permanently. Talk to your program director or advisor about what programs or groups are available to help you quit.

And, remember, teaming up with classmates for support to quit can be exactly the encouragement you both need.

Avoid sugary or high calorie snacks while studying. Stick to regular, healthy mealtimes, and plan for needed snacks by having fruit, vegetable sticks, small portions of low-fat, high protein food available.

Take a break for 5 to 10 minutes after each 50 minutes of study. The following are suggestions:

Stand and stretch

Walk around; get some fresh air

Drink a glass of water

Shake your arms and tell your fingers, hands, and arms to relax

Raise and lower your shoulders and tell your shoulders to relax

TEST-TAKING STRATEGIES FOR MULTIPLE CHOICE TESTS:

1. Read the test instructions carefully, first. Note whether there is a time limit and plan quickly the amount of time to spend on each section of the text.
2. Scan the entire question.
3. Read the body of the question again and consider what it is asking.
4. Read each option.
5. Eliminate all unlikely options.
6. Look at remaining options and eliminate options with any wrong or inconsistent statements.

Hints:

Watch for statements in the body of the question or the options, in which one word changes the meaning of the statement: NOT, EXCEPT, NEVER, ONLY, ALWAYS

Look closely at options that are longer or much shorter than the others—these are either definitely the wrong or right answer

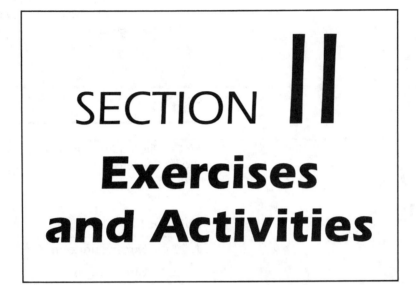

SECTION II
Exercises and Activities

1

The Origins of Nursing

✪ Be sure to review the Learning Objectives from the text.

✔ Be sure to FIRST perform Improving Concentration exercises described in Section One before proceeding with the next exercise.

Part 1

Match the headings in column I with the major headings in this chapter under which they may be found in column II.

Column I

1. _____ Nursing uniforms
2. _____ Early influences
3. _____ Florence Nightingale
4. _____ Nursing during wartimes
5. _____ The Reformation

Column II

a. Nursing's Heritage

b. Nursing in the United States

c. Nursing Insignia

Common Acronyms or Terms

AIDS	NCLEX
AJN	NFLPN
AMA	NLN
ANA	NSNA
HOSA	RN
ICN	VNS
LPN	YMCA
LVN	YWCA
NAPNES	

Part 2

Read the key points, then answer the following statements true (T) or false (F) and correct the false statements.

1. _____ The first practical nursing school in the United States opened in 1892 in New Jersey.

2. _____ Nursing insignia, such as those found on nursing school pins, often symbolize nursing's future and heritage.

3. _____ Medicine men and women and religious orders cared for the sick in early times.

4. _____ Establishment of nursing schools in the United States began in the late 18th century.

5. _____ Florence Nightingale contributed a great deal to the development of contemporary nursing.

CHAPTER OVERVIEW

Chapter 1 discusses nursing's early beginnings, its progression and influences in the United States, and the insignia associated with nursing.

Part 3

Associate the terms from column I to a term in column II.

Column I

1. _____ Crimean War
2. _____ Roman matron
3. _____ Student progress record
4. _____ Father of medicine
5. _____ First geriatric facility
6. _____ Crusades
7. _____ Symbol of Nightingale School
8. _____ Site of Nightingale School
9. _____ 1500
10. _____ Greek hostels
11. _____ Nightingale's alma mater
12. _____ First nonhospital nursing school

Column II

a. About 500 B.C.

b. Male military nurses/knights

c. Dark ages of nursing

d. St. Thomas Hospital, London

e. 1860

f. Kaiserwerth School of Nursing

g. Lady with the lamp

h. Hippocratic Oath

i. Fabiola

j. Maltese cross

k. Nightingale plan

l. St. Helena

Part 4

Use the information under the heading of Nursing in the United States to answer the following questions. Number the terms in order from the most recent being number 1 to the most historical being number 12.

_____ NLN publishes entry level competencies of graduates from LPN/LVN programs.

_____ New York becomes first state to mandate licensure of practical nurses.

_____ Isabel Robb founds *American Journal of Nursing*.

_____ Pittsburgh Infirmary begins training nurses in the United States.

_____ First computerized exam, NCLEX, is given for nursing licensure.

_____ Clara Barton founds American Red Cross.

_____ University of Minnesota is first school to educate nurses at university level.

_____ All states now have laws to license practical nurses.

_____ Lillian Wald founds Visiting Nurses Association.

_____ Mississippi becomes the first state to license practical nurses.

_____ NLN accredits the first practical nursing program.

_____ Linda Richards becomes the first trained nurse in the United States.

2

Beginning Your Nursing Career

Common Acronyms or Terms

AALPN	CNA	NCLEX-PN
AD	e-mail	NLN-CHAP
ANCC	INC	UAP

CHAPTER OVERVIEW

Chapter 2 discusses various programs for nursing education, approval, accreditation, and licensure. The code of ethics, the role and image of the nurse, and nursing organizations are also discussed.

✪ Be sure to review the Learning Objectives from the text.

✔ Be sure to FIRST perform Improving Concentration exercises described in Section One before proceeding with the next exercise.

Part 1

Complete the following statements related to the major headings in this chapter.

1. The two headings under the major category of "Types of Nursing Programs" identify that the nursing programs discussed prepare their graduates to become either a _____ or _____ _____ nurse.

2. The second major heading indicates that nursing programs may be _____ or _____ by a nursing authority or nursing agency such as the National League for Nursing.

3. Name two organizations listed under the heading "Nursing Organizations": _____ and _____.

Part 2

Read the key points at the end of the chapter, then indicate with a T for true or F for false which of the following is a true or false statement.

1. ____ One type of nursing education is available that leads to licensure as a registered nurse (RN) or as a licensed practical nurse (LPN)/licensed vocational nurse (LVN).

2. ____ Nurses promise to practice ethically when they recite pledges at graduation.

3. ____ Hospitals are the agencies that set standards of practice for RNs and for LPNs.

Part 3 Key Terms: Knowledge Check

Review the key terms in the chapter. Mark (y) beside the terms you know the definition of and (n) beside the terms you do not know. List the terms marked with an (n) in the spaces below and write the definition of each as you read.

Term

_____

_____

_____

_____

Definition

_____

_____

_____

_____

Part 4

Fill in the spaces with the terms defined below them.

1. _____
   The law does not forbid practicing nursing without a license but forbids the use of the title LPN/LVN or RN.

2. _____ Nurse
   An RN usually with a master's degree who has specialized in a particular field

3. _____
   A skeleton on which to hang knowledge; provides a basis for forming a personal philosophy of nursing.

Part 5 Short Answer and Completions

Complete the following fill-in-the-blank exercises.

1. Defining the specific roles of a nurse is _____
   _____ because these roles constantly _____.

2. The type of nurse assigned to a client usually depends on the degree of the individual's _____
   _____.

3. A program can be _____ by the state's Board of Nursing without being _____
   _____ by a national organization such as the National League for Nursing.

4. The common roles of the nurse include nurse as care provider, communicator, advocate,
   _____, _____,
   and _____ _____.

Part 6

Indicate if the statement is accurate for LPN/LVN or for RN practice by placing the appropriate initials in front of the statement.

1. _____ Most nursing programs exist under the auspices of a public education unit such as a community college.

2. _____ Must attend a 2-, 3-, or 4-year nursing program leading to licensure.

3. _____ Must practice under the direction of another healthcare person such as a physician.

Part 7. Multiple Choice

Circle the letter corresponding to the correct answer.

1. Nursing practice standards for the LPN/LVN include which of the following?
   a. Education standards stating that the LPN/LVN must complete an accredited nursing program
   b. Practice standards stating that the LPN/LVN may function independently in caring for clients
   c. Legal/ethical standards stating that the LPN/LVN shall take responsible actions in situations wherein there is unprofessional conduct by a peer or other healthcare provider
   d. Continuing education standards stating that LPNs/LVNs should attend a program preparing for RN practice within 1 year of being licensed

2. Virginia Henderson is a nursing theorist whose model of practice was:
   a. Self-care
   b. Natural healing
   c. Systems
   d. Independent functioning

3. National organizations whose membership include the LPN/LVN include all of the following except the:
   a. ANA
   b. AALPN
   c. NAPNES
   d. NLN-CHAP

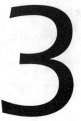

Healthcare Delivery System

Common Acronyms or Terms

CQI

DRG

ECF

HMO

HPRDA

ICF

IHS

JCAHO

OSHA

PPO

RUG

SSDI

CHAPTER OVERVIEW

Chapter 3 discusses healthcare in the 21st century and the changing roles of nurses. Healthcare reform and holistic healthcare are discussed. The settings for healthcare are also discussed.

✪ Be sure to review the Learning Objectives from the text.

✔ Be sure to FIRST perform Improving Concentration exercises described in Section One before proceeding with the next exercise.

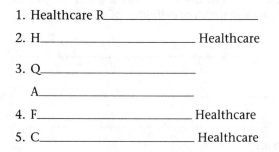

Part 1

Complete the following titles found as major headings in this chapter.

1. Healthcare R_____

2. H_____ Healthcare

3. Q_____

    A_____

4. F_____ Healthcare

5. C_____ Healthcare

Part 2

Complete the following statements related to the major headings and key concepts.

1. Two of the headings under the major heading "Settings for Healthcare" include _____ _____ and _____.

2. Holism is a philosophy that views the _____ _____ person.

Part 3. Key Terms: Knowledge Check

Review the key terms in the chapter. Mark (y) beside the terms you recognize and can define and (n) beside the terms you do not know. List the terms marked with an (n) in the spaces below and write an abbreviated definition of each term as you read.

Term

_____

_____

_____

_____

Definition

_____

_____

_____

_____

_____

Part 4

Fill in term or terms that best match(es) the definition.

1. _____
   To assist the client and family to make hospitalization as comfortable and free of stress as possible

2. _____
   Joint effort of federal and state governments, generally for people over 65, blind, disabled, or AFDC

3. _____
   Misleading the public, illegal

4. _____
   Payment made in advance to HMO, participant then entitled to healthcare without further charge (except for predetermined co-pay)

5. _____
   Requires objective and systematic monitoring and evaluation of the quality and appropriateness of client care

Part 5

Answer these statements true (T) or false (F).

1. _____ The information you are learning about healthcare today will not change for several years to come.

2. _____ The primary role of the hospital is to provide education.

3. _____ The public spends an estimated $25 billion on "sure cures," some of which are fraudulent.

4. _____ Holistic healthcare defines health in terms of the underlying disease.

5. _____ The term "patient" implies participation in decision-making regarding one's own health.

6. _____ Medicare is available to nearly everyone over 65, no matter what their financial status.

7. _____ Quality control and quality assurance focus on how well the clients receive the care offered to them.

8. _____ Therapeutic touch uses the energy (electromagnetic) field around each person.

9. _____ Telehealth is the ability to access a nurse via television videotape.

10. _____ Insurance companies may refuse to insure people they consider high risk.

Part 6

Match the contemporary healthcare concepts in column I with their definition in column II.

Column I

1. _____ Teaches skills enabling self-care

2. _____ Concentration to allow relaxation of all muscle groups

3. _____ Use of mental picture to treat cancer and other chronic conditions

4. _____ Manipulation of spinal column and joints to treat pain and discomfort

5. _____ External pressure applied to energy points

6. _____ Rehabilitation important in the management of chronic disorders

7. _____ Also considered a healing meditation

8. _____ Insertion of fine needles into energy points

9. _____ Promoting health using flower essences

10. _____ Thought and breath control that helps to decrease anxiety and help people to cope with stress

Column II

a. Acupressure

b. Therapeutic touch

c. Meditation

d. Occupational therapy

e. Vibrational remedies

f. Chiropractic

g. Imagery

h. Therapeutic relaxation

i. Physical therapy

j. Acupuncture

Part 7. Short Answer Exercises

List two of the commonalities between the pairs listed below.

1. DRGs — RUGs

2. Medicare — Medicaid

3. SNF — ICF

4

Legal and Ethical Aspects of Nursing

Common Acronyms or Terms

AHA

AMA

CEU

CNS

NAHC

NCLEX-RN

PSDA

UNOS

CHAPTER OVERVIEW

Chapter 4 discusses the laws and regulations governing nursing practice and ethical standards in healthcare. The nurse's legal and ethical responsibilities and legal rights are reviewed related to nursing practice. Legal issues and ethical problems in healthcare are addressed.

✪ Be sure to review the Learning Objectives from the text.

✔ Be sure to FIRST perform Improving Concentration exercises described in Section One before proceeding with the next exercise.

Part 1

Indicate the order in which you find the following major headings in this chapter.

1. _____ Legal Responsibilities in Nursing

2. _____ Values Clarification

3. _____ Regulations of Nursing Practice

4. _____ Ethical Standards of Healthcare

Part 2

Complete the following statements related to the major headings and key points.

1. A nurse is _____ and _____ bound to practice nursing within the rules and regulations of your Nursing Practice Act and within the laws of your state, territory, or province.

2. The last major heading found in this chapter (after "Values Clarification") is _____.

Part 3 Key Terms: Knowledge Check

Review the key terms in the chapter. Mark (y) beside the terms you recognize and can define and (n) beside the terms you do not know. List the terms marked with an (n) in the spaces below and write an abbreviated definition of each term as you read.

Term

_____

_____

_____

_____

Definition

_____

_____

_____

_____

_____

Copyright © 1999 Lippincott Williams & Wilkins, **Study Guide to Accompany Caroline Bunker Rosdahl's Textbook of Basic Nursing, Seventh Edition** by Joyce Young Johnson and Phyllis Prather-Hicks

Part 4

Fill in term or terms that best match(es) the definition.

1. _____
   A written and legally witnessed document that requests no extraordinary measures to be taken to save a person's life in the event of terminal illness

2. _____
   Deliberate taking of a person's life to put the individual out of their misery; called "mercy killing"

3. _____
   The legal responsibility for one's actions or failure to act appropriately

4. _____
   A violent act, either physical or verbal

5. _____
   Client permission given after the tests, treatments, and medications have been explained to the person, as well as outcomes, possible complications, and alternative procedures

Part 5

Answer these statements true (T) or false (F).

1. _____ A tort is a wrong committed against another person or property.

2. _____ The laws in all states are consistent and indicate that assisted suicide is illegal.

3. _____ A client has the responsibility to follow the recommended treatment plan.

4. _____ The Patient Self-Determination Act (PSDA) states that terminally ill individuals must sign an advance directive when admitted to a healthcare institution.

5. _____ A nurse should accept personal gifts from clients because refusing the gift might offend the person.

Part 6

Match the definitions in column I with the contemporary healthcare concepts in column II.

Column I

1. _____ A physical striking or beating

2. _____ A crime punishable by law, such as presenting false documents to an employer

3. _____ Malicious verbal statements that are false or injurious

4. _____ A legal document in which a person either states choices for medical treatment or names someone to make treatment choices if he or she loses decision-making ability

5. _____ A serious crime, such as stealing a client's money or murder

6. _____ Written statement or photograph that is false or damaging

7. _____ A wrong committed against a person or property and also the public good as mandated by law

8. _____ Consciously examining your own values, beliefs, and feelings about life and healthcare issues

9. _____ Conduct appropriate for all members of a group

10. _____ Clinical death also known as irreversible coma

Column II

a. Values clarification

b. Advance directives

c. Brain death

d. Crime

e. Battery

f. Slander

g. Ethics

h. Libel

i. Fraud

j. Felony

Part 7. Short Answer Exercises

Complete the following short answer questions.

1. What are important considerations for the nurse in maintaining professional boundaries? _____

   _____

2. Name two advance directives other than a living will. _____

   _____

3. State two type of adult individuals who would be considered vulnerable adults. _____

   _____

5

Basic Human Needs

Common Acronyms or Terms

CHD	MI
COPD	MUA
HDL	STD
HIV	WHO

CHAPTER OVERVIEW

Chapter 5 discusses Maslow's hierarchy of basic needs. An overview of individual, family, and community needs is provided with examination of the relationship between nursing care and the basic and higher needs of individuals.

✪ Be sure to review the Learning Objectives from the text.

✔ Be sure to FIRST perform Improving Concentration exercises described in Section One before proceeding with the next exercise.

Part 1

Complete the following titles found as major headings in this chapter.

1. Maslow's H_____ of Needs

2. Nursing's R_____ to Basic

   _____

3. F_____ and C_____ Needs

Part 2

Complete the following statements related to the major headings and key concepts.

1. Three of the headings under the major heading "Basic Physiologic Needs" include _____, _____, and _____.

2. The need for freedom from harm and for shelter fall under the heading of _____ and _____ needs.

Part 3 Matching of Key Terms: Knowledge Check

Match the following key terms in the chapter with the appropriate definition.

Column I

1. _____ Aesthetic needs

2. _____ Homeostasis

3. _____ Regression

4. _____ Secondary needs

5. _____ Self-actualized

Column II

a. When an individual has reached his or her full potential

b. Needs that are met to give quality to life

c. The more complex human needs

d. Focusing on a lower level need that has already been fulfilled

e. Balance maintained in the fluids in the body to maintain health

Part 4

Fill in term or terms that best match(es) the definition.

1. _____
   A ladder on which needs are ranked by their importance to the individual's survival

2. _____
   A basic physiologic need that may be sublimated; vital to the survival of the species

3. _____

   Basic survival needs common to all animals, including human beings

4. _____

   Love and belonging needs; people must meet survival and security needs before addressing these

Part 5

Indicate on which level of the Hierarchy of Needs pyramid the following needs are found.

1. _____ Self-esteem needs

2. _____ Freedom from harm

3. _____ Spiritual needs

4. _____ Water and fluids

5. _____ Warmth

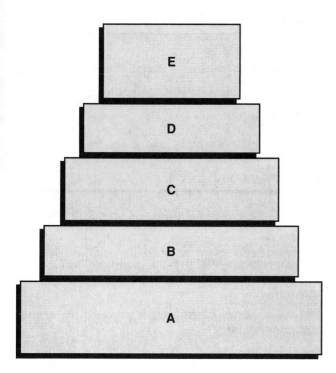

6

Health and Wellness

Common Acronyms or Terms

CHD

COPD

HDL

HIV

LDL

MI

MVA

STD

WHO

CHAPTER OVERVIEW

Chapter 6 explores the definitions of wellness, health, and illness. Health concerns related to persons in various age groups are discussed. Health goals for the nation are discussed with emphasis on health promotion. Measures for promoting behavior change to healthy living are also addressed.

❂ Be sure to review the Learning Objectives from the text.

✔ Be sure to FIRST perform Improving Concentration exercises described in Section One before proceeding with the next exercise.

Part 1

Match the headings in column I with the major headings in this chapter under which they may be found in column II.

Column I

1. _____ Stress

2. _____ Categories of Deviation from Normal

3. _____ Education

4. _____ Violence and Abuse

5. _____ Children and Adolescents

6. _____ Nutrition

Column II

a. Keys to Changing Behavior

b. Health Promotion and Lifestyle Factors

c. Health Concerns Related to Age Groups

d. Health, Illness, and Wellness

Part 2

Fill in term or terms that best match(es) the definition.

1. _____
   A process in which tumor cells spread to other parts of the body

2. _____
   Loss of bone density that is prevalent in women; causes fractures

3. _____
   The "wear and tear" of life—physical and psychological factors that interfere with homeostasis

4. _____
   Used to prevent cholesterol from collecting in arteries, reduce heart disease, and retard aging

5. _____
   Can contribute dramatically to improvement of overall health and reduced deaths

Part 3

Match the following health concerns in column I with the age groups listed in column II.

Column I

1. _____ Heart disease

2. _____ Respiratory distress syndrome

3. _____ Suicide

4. _____ Sexually transmitted diseases

5. _____ Osteoporosis

Column II

a. Infants

b. Children and adolescents

c. Adult women

d. Adult men

Part 4 Short Answer Exercises

Complete the following short answer questions.

1. Briefly discuss the benefit of four lifestyle factors in improving health and reducing death.

   _____

   _____

   _____

   _____

   _____

2. Discuss prevention measures that the nurse might implement to promote: a healthy pregnancy, a decrease in cancer.

   _____

   _____

   _____

   _____

   _____

Part 5 Multiple Choice

Circle the letter corresponding to the correct answer.

1. Peter Lawson, age 19, is admitted for repair of a heart condition that he was born with because his mother contracted German measles during her pregnancy with him. The heart condition would be considered a:
   a. Metabolic disorder causing a functional disease
   b. Congenital disorder causing an organic disease
   c. Hereditary disorder causing a functional disease
   d. Traumatic disorder causing an organic disease

2. The body adapts to change to:
   a. Maintain homeostasis
   b. Establish high-level wellness
   c. Maintain optimal health
   d. Establish self-actualization

3. Which of the following statements is true regarding lifestyle factors?
   a. Physical activity is not effective for managing chronic illnesses such as arthritis.
   b. Poor nutrition contributes to congestive heart failure, cancer, and obesity.
   c. Laws regulating substance use are effectively enforced to decrease drug use.
   d. Rape and other sexual crimes are reported less frequently today than in past years.

4. Tobacco use:
   a. Is not dangerous if the smokeless form is used
   b. Results in dilatation of the arteries and a decreased heart rate
   c. Has lifelong effects that cannot be reversed by smoking cessation
   d. May aggravate conditions including periodontal disease or osteoporosis

5. Health promotion and disease prevention measures include which of the following?
   a. Instructing the client with a risk for cancer to follow a high-fat diet to decrease risk
   b. Informing the public that prevention of heart attack includes a low-protein diet
   c. Decreasing physical activity in persons with hypertension to lower blood pressure
   d. Helping clients with diabetes to manage their weight and follow dietary guidelines

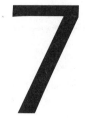

Community Health

Common Acronyms or Terms

ACS	MHA
ADA	MUA
AHA	NIH
ARC	NIOSH
ATF	OMH
BOH	OTC
CDC	TTY
DOA	UN
DOH	UNICEF
FDA	USDHHS
FQHC	USPHS
HRA	VNA
HSA	WIC
MCHB	

CHAPTER OVERVIEW

Chapter 7 discusses the health concerns of an entire population and implications for the nurse. Healthcare on the local level, state level, and national level is addressed with an overview of the various organizations involved in providing community health services. Healthcare worldwide and environmental impacts on community health are also discussed.

✪ Be sure to review the Learning Objectives from the text.

✤ Be sure to FIRST perform Improving Concentration exercises described in the Introduction before proceeding with the next exercise.

Part 1

Indicate the order in which you find the following major headings in this chapter.

_____ The Environment

_____ Healthcare on the National Level

_____ Healthcare Worldwide

_____ Health in the Community

_____ Healthcare on the State Level

Part 2

Complete the following statements related to the major headings and key points.

1. A nurse is a member of many communities and should serve as an (a) _____ and a _____ to protect those communities.

2. United Nations programs and communicable disease control are headings under the major heading of H_____ W_____.

Part 3 Key Terms: Knowledge Check

Review the key terms in the chapter. Mark (y) beside the terms you recognize and can define and (n) beside the terms you do not know. List the terms marked with an (n) in the spaces below and write an abbreviated definition of each term as you read.

Term

_____

_____

_____

_____

_____

Definition

_____

_____

_____

_____

_____

Part 4

Fill in term or terms that best match(es) the definition.

1. _____
   Medical waste that is harmful to humans or animals; infectious

2. _____
   The study of mutual relationships between living beings and their environment; bionomics

3. _____
   Lead poisoning that can cause serious disabilities, particularly in young children

4. _____
   Collaboration between public and private organizations who share data and workers to provide more cost-effective healthcare

5. _____
   Family-focused healthcare that emphasizes health education and wellness to promote healthy lifestyles and decrease the potential for illness

Part 5

Answer these statements true (T) or false (F).

1. _____ Health departments provide services to specific residents in the community with a limited number of conditions.

2. _____ In some areas, local and state health departments now refer clients to private providers through Medicaid or charity care programs.

3. _____ Worker's compensation is one form of healthcare on the local level.

4. _____ Proper and safe disposal of biohazardous medical wastes is the responsibility of the state agencies and local health department, not the institutional or individual healthcare provider.

5. _____ Disputes between the public and power companies using nuclear fuel concern the disposal of radioactive wastes.

Part 6

Match the agency responsibilities in column I with the agency names listed in column II.

Column I

1. _____ Inspects work sites and makes recommendations to protect workers and students from job-related injuries and illnesses

2. _____ Established in an attempt to control problems relating to the ecology

3. _____ Carries out policies and regulations under the direction of a health officer; inspect food places

4. _____ Analyzes causes of accidents and suggests preventive measures

5. _____ Duties include investigation and control of communicable diseases and control of sanitation

Column II

a. Environmental Protection Agency

b. Occupational Safety and Health Administration

c. National Safety Council

d. United States Public Health Service

e. Department of Health

Part 7 Multiple Choice Exercises

Circle the letter corresponding to the correct answer.

1. You have a client who has infected rat bites and states that the entire apartment complex is infested. You would appropriately notify which of the following agencies?
   a. The Food and Drug Administration
   b. The Social Security Administration
   c. The Department of Agriculture
   d. The American Red Cross

2. The community health center in your area has hired you to assist with projects during the summer. You would expect that your duties might include:
   a. Arranging times for all families served by this center to come to the central office so that care can be given in one location
   b. Working with clients in group homes for the mentally ill or retarded, day care centers, or in school settings

c. Referring clients with suspected sexually transmitted diseases (STDs) to a hospital for screening

d. Scheduling clients for visits to the the emergency room to receive immunizations and prenatal care

3. Encouraging families to obtain and use a radon testing kit would help to prevent disease related to which of the following?
   a. Water pollution
   b. Land pollution
   c. Noise pollution
   d. Air pollution

8

Transcultural Healthcare

Common Acronyms or Terms

LDS   RC

CHAPTER OVERVIEW

Chapter 8 discusses the issue of culture and ethnicity and the impact of these issues on healthcare delivery. Barriers to culturally competent nursing care are addressed. Common culturally influenced components are reviewed and culturally competent care is discussed.

✪ Be sure to review the Learning Objectives from the text.

✔ Be sure to FIRST perform Improving Concentration exercises described in the Introduction before proceeding with the next exercise.

Part 1

*Which of the following major headings is **not** located in this chapter. Place a "Y" by those in the chapter and an "N" by those not in the chapter.*

_____ Culture and Ethnicity

_____ Culturally Influenced Components

_____ Healthcare Worldwide

_____ Religious/Spiritual Customs and Traditions

_____ Implementing Culturally Competent Care

Part 2

Complete the following statements related to the major headings and key points.

1. Cultural and religious traditions are _____ _____ followed by every member of a group. (Always/Not always)

2. Values and beliefs, health and illness, and taboos and rituals are under the major heading of: C _ _ _ _ _ _ _ _ I _ _ _ _ _ _ _ _ C _ _ _ _ _ _ _ _

Part 3 Key Terms: Knowledge Check

Review the key terms in the chapter. Mark the following statements with T for true or F for false to indicate the accuracy of these statements.

1. _____ Cultural diversity is rare in the United States.

2. _____ Prejudice is an impression formed about a person after detailed examination.

3. _____ Ethnocentrism is the belief that one's own culture is best and is the only acceptable way.

4. _____ You can deliver culturally competent care without developing cultural sensitivity.

5. _____ Cultures have taboos that members cannot violate without discomfort.

Part 4

Fill in term or terms that best match(es) the definition.

1. _____
   Members are required to practice these for comfort, acceptance, and inclusion

2. _____
   Concepts that the members of the group feel are true

3. _____
   To classify or categorize people, believing that all those people of a certain group are alike

4. _____
   Ethnic-sensitive nursing care

Part 5

Match the statement in column I with the closely related term or concept in column II.

Column I

1. _____ Some groups are magicoreligious and feel that healing will occur with prayer alone; others groups feel the forces of nature must be kept balanced for health.

2. _____ Unified opposites that are interrelated; a "cold" illness requires a "hot" treatment.

3. _____ A person's comfort zone; some cultures maintain a distance of several feet apart for comfort.

4. _____ Looking at another person; can give important cues about clients because such action is culturally influenced.

5. _____ A vital part of many people's lives; includes Christianity, Judaism, and Islam.

Column II

a. Religion

b. Personal space

c. Yin and Yang

d. Health belief systems

e. Eye contact

Part 6 Multiple Choice Exercises

Circle the letter corresponding to the correct answer.

1. Tashah Michai, age 16, is of East Indian culture, and is scheduled for a physical examination. The doctor, Dr. Fred Reed, enters and asks you to prepare for a pelvic examination and Pap smear. You notice Tashah seems very nervous and her mother and father state they must take Tashah home now. You would:
   a. Tell Tashah and her parents to calm down and explain the procedure.
   b. Ask Tashah and her parents if they were uneasy about having a male doctor examine Tashah.
   c. Inform Tashah and her parents that a Pap smear should be done because Tashah is now a young woman.
   d. Tell Dr. Reed that Tashah and her parents seem to be nervous and uncomfortable and ask him to speak with them.

2. Norah Vorna was admitted to your unit last week with end-stage cancer. A new nurse comes to you and complains that the Vorna family is in the room with an electric candelabra. You would explain that:
   a. If the Vorna family has received special permission to use this electrical device, they may use it to exercise their cultural practices.
   b. Candles of any sort are forbidden in a hospital setting so the nurse should go back to the room and ask them to take the candelabra home.
   c. The nurse is responsible for making sure families follow hospital procedures so the nurse should suggest that the Vorna family perform these rituals after the client is discharged.
   d. The nurse should wait until the family leaves and remove the candelabra and take it to hospital security.

3. You are expecting a new client admission to your unit. You are informed that he is a 40-year-old Chinese American who has been in this country with his family for 20 years. You would act based on which of the following understandings about language and communication?
   a. Professional interpreters are not needed if the client has been in the United States more than 10 years.
   b. A family member is the best person to act as an interpreter because he or she will keep findings confidential.
   c. An interpreter might be needed even if the client previously communicated well because many people regress when ill.
   d. A bilingual healthcare worker should be sought because there is no problem having the healthcare worker to serve as an interpreter for any client in their hospital setting.

4. You discover that your postoperative surgery client, Mr. Cohen, is eating only the fruits and bread on the food tray. The record states that he practices Orthodox Judaism. You would:
   a. Stress the importance of nutritional intake with Mr. Cohen and his family.
   b. Explore Mr. Cohen's preferences and ask dietary to place meat and dairy products in separate dishes.
   c. Insist that Mr. Cohen eat his pork chops because the protein will help him heal.
   d. Tell dietary to provide larger portions of fruit and bread and praise Mr. Cohen for eating all of these two food servings.

9

The Family

Common Acronyms or Terms

SO

CHAPTER OVERVIEW

Chapter 9 discusses various aspects of the family. Family structure is addressed with an overview of different types of families. Family stages are discussed in addition to the stress families encounter and coping mechanisms used.

✪ Be sure to review the Learning Objectives from the text

✔ Be sure to FIRST perform Improving Concentration exercises described in the Introduction before proceeding with the next exercise.

Part 1

Indicate the order in which you find the following major headings and subheadings in this chapter.

_____ Family Violence

_____ Family Structure

_____ Effective and Ineffective Coping Strategies

_____ Stress and Family Coping

_____ Socioeconomic Stressors

_____ Family Stages

Part 2

Complete the following statements related to the major headings and key points.

1. The family is the basic unit of society, but it is a _____ unit.

2. Two of the three "family stages" listed under that heading are _____ and _____ stage.

3. Culture, _____, and _____ factors influence family outcomes.

Part 3 Key Terms: Knowledge Check

Review the key terms in the chapter. Mark (y) beside the terms you recognize and can define and (n) beside the terms you do not know. List the terms marked with an (n) in the spaces below and write an abbreviated definition of each term as you read.

Term

_____

_____

_____

_____

Definition

_____

_____

_____

_____

Part 4

Fill in term or terms to indicate the type of family described.

1. _____
   Consists of the nuclear family and other related persons such as grandparents, aunts, and cousins

2. _____
   A family in which a divorce or separation occurs

but both parents continue to assume a high level of childrearing responsibilities

3. _____

Involves an adult head of the house with dependent children; may result from divorce, or death

4. _____

A two-generation unit consisting of a husband, wife, and their immediate children living within one household

Part 5

Answer these statements true (T) or false (F).

1. _____ A transitional stage refers to the period when single young adults are financially independent from their family or origin and live outside the family home.

2. _____ In the expanding family stage, child launching, postparenting, and aging are concerns.

3. _____ Reconstituted families are those in which the parents have rededicated themselves to each other and the children after a separation.

4. _____ Dual-career families are those in which both parents work outside the home.

5. _____ A nuclear dyad is a family in which there are two children, one male and one female.

Part 6

Match the definitions in column I with the family concepts in column II.

Column I

1. _____ An adult living alone in their own apartment or house

2. _____ The family has reached maximum size; begins as the first child leaves home to live independently

3. _____ Families that cannot cope; stressors build and coping systems disintegrate

4. _____ Single adults move into the this phase when they choose a partner and set up a household.

5. _____ Begins when the youngest child leaves home and continues until the retirement or death of a partner

6. _____ Unmarried individuals in a committed partnership living together, with or without children

Column II

a. Establishment

b. Dysfunctional families

c. Postparenting

d. Cohabitation

e. Single adult household

f. Child launching

Part 7 Short Answer Exercises

Complete the following short answer questions.

1. Indicate three sources of stress a family may encounter.

   _____

   _____

2. State two types of alternative families.

   _____

   _____

Part 8

Indicate if the following are effective (E) or ineffective (I) coping patterns.

1. _____ Recognizing that stress is temporary and may be positive

2. _____ Feeling a sense of accomplishment in dealing with stress

3. _____ Focusing on family problems rather than strengths

4. _____ Developing new rules for changing situations

5. _____ Growing to dislike family life as a result of accumulation of stress

10

Infancy and Childhood

CHAPTER OVERVIEW

Chapter 10 presents an overview of human growth and development from infancy through childhood. Physical growth as well as psychosocial development and cognitive and motor development are discussed. Growth and development theories, areas of concern, and anticipatory guidance are addressed.

✪ Be sure to review the Learning Objectives from the text.

✔ Be sure to FIRST perform Improving Concentration exercises described in the Introduction before proceeding with the next exercise.

Part 1

Complete the following statements related to the major headings in this chapter.

1. The headings under the major category of "Growth and Development" identify the 'concepts of', 'influences on', and theories of growth and development, in addition, the role of _____ in child development and _____ _____ are discussed.

2. The second major heading of the chapter discusses the N_ _ _ _ _ _.

3. Complete the title of the major headings for the chapter listed below by indicating the age range for the growth and development stages:

Infancy: _____ to _____ months

Toddlerhood: _____ to _____ years

Preschool: _____ to _____ years

School age: _____ to _____ years

Part 2

Read the key points at the end of the chapter, then indicate with a T for true or F for false which of the following is a true or false statement.

1. _____ Preschool is the period of fastest growth and development over the entire life span.

2. _____ Play helps prepare children for more mature levels of functioning.

3. _____ Nurses can give anticipatory guidance to help prepare family caregivers for the normal areas of concern that arise during each developmental stage.

Part 3 Key Terms: Knowledge Check

Match the terms in column I with the definitions in column II.

Column I

1. _____ Bonding
2. _____ Cognitive
3. _____ Development
4. _____ Environment
5. _____ Enuresis
6. _____ Proximodistal
7. _____ Hereditary
8. _____ Masturbation
9. _____ Regression
10. _____ Growth

Column II

a. Characteristics that are often called genetic factors, such as eye color and body build

b. The sum of all the conditions and factors surrounding the child, such as housing, siblings

c. Attachment to parents and other family caregivers

d. The handling and self-stimulation of the genital organs

e. Knowledge, understanding, or perception; the process of thinking

f. A change in body size and structure

g. Bed-wetting

h. A change in body function

i. Behavior that goes backward to that of an earlier stage of development

j. From the center to the outside; babies roll over before they grasp small objects.

Part 4

Fill in the spaces with the letters of terms defined below. The first letter is provided.

1. O_ _ _ _ _ _ P_ _ _ _ _ _ _ _ _
The knowledge that an object seen in a particular spot but temporarily hidden from view under a blanket continues to exist and will return to view when it is uncovered

2. I _ _ _ _ _ _ _ _ _ _ _ _ _ _ _
All aspects of growth and development relate to other aspects; control of bowel movements cannot occur until muscles are strong enough and child understands expectations.

3. C _ _ _ _ _ _ _ _ _ _ _ _ _ _ _
Means from head to tail; for example, babies lift their heads before they sit up.

Part 5 Short Answer and Completions

Complete the following fill-in-the-blank exercises.

1. Havighurst theorizes that each life stage has its own group of developmental _ _ _ _ _ that a person

must accomplish to become a mature, fully functioning individual.

2. Most providers agree that solids should not be introduced into the diet before infants reach _____ months of age.

3. Discuss the condition known as nursing bottle mouth including the definition of the phrase, common causes, and associated problems that might be experienced. _____

4. Toddlers need simple, consistent guidance; therefore, families must begin to establish l_ _ _ _ s_ _ _ _ _ for children at this stage.

5. Sibling rivalry, phobias and nightmares, masturbation, and enuresis are areas of concern for the _____ stage child.

Part 6

For 1. and 2., indicate the appropriate order in which the following stages of development occur:

1. Erikson's stages of psychosocial development

_____ autonomy vs shame and doubt

_____ initiative vs guilt

_____ trust vs mistrust

_____ industry vs inferiority

2. Piaget: stages of cognitive development

_____ formal operations

_____ preoperations

_____ sensorimotor

_____ concrete operations

3. The school-age child should have some tasks to do in the home, such as cleaning the bedroom or loading the dishwasher, because these tasks allow the child to acquire a sense of _____.

11

Adolescence

CHAPTER OVERVIEW

Chapter 11 addresses the physical, psychosocial, emotional, cognitive, and moral development of adolescence. Theories of growth and development are discussed in relationship to the adolescent. An overview of areas of concern in adolescent development is provided.

✪ Be sure to review the Learning Objectives from the text.

✍ Be sure to FIRST perform Improving Concentration exercises described in the Introduction before proceeding with the next exercise.

Part 1

Complete the following titles and statements found as major headings and key points in this chapter.

1. Havighurst, Erikson, and Piaget are discussed under which major heading in this chapter: G _ _ _ _ _ and D_ _ _ _ _ _ _ _ _ _ T _ _ _ _ _ _ _ .

2. The heading "Adolescent Growth and Development" contains subheadings that include: physical growth, psychosocial development, areas of concern, and c_ _ _ _ _ _ _ _, e _ _ _ _ _ _ _ _, and m _ _ _ _ development.

3. P _ _ _ _ _ _ is the time when a person matures sexually and becomes able to reproduce.

4. Great v_ _ _ _ _ _ _ _ exists in physical and emotional maturity among young people.

Part 2 Matching Key Terms: Knowledge Check

Match the following key terms in the chapter with the appropriate definition.

Column I

1. _____ Menarche
2. _____ Nocturnal emission
3. _____ Preadolescence
4. _____ Peer group
5. _____ Adolescence

Column II

a. Involuntary discharge of semen while sleeping; a normal part of male reproductive health

b. Made up of contemporaries or people with whom the adolescent associates

c. The onset of menstruation; usually occurs by age 13

d. The developmental period between puberty and maturity

e. An early "awkward" stage, pubescence; lasts from ages 11 to 14 years

Part 3

Indicate which theorist proposed which of the following concepts. Use E for Erikson, P for Piaget, and H for Havighurst.

1. _____ The ultimate task of adolescence is to 'grow up' and includes such activities as achieving emotional independence.

2. _____ Adolescents face challenges with personal identity versus role confusion, and develop virtues that include independence, self-esteem, self-reliance, self-control, devotion, and fidelity.

3. _____ Skill development is part of cognitive growth and is also preparation for the future.

4. _____ The adolescent aged 12 to 15 years enters the cognitive development stage of formal operations in which one thinks in the abstract and does complex problem-solving.

5. _____ Tasks of adolescence include preparation for a career, education, and other pursuits.

Part 4

Circle the letter corresponding to the correct answer.

1. Jane Parker has brought her son Mike, age 12, to the hospital. She states he has informed her that he has a crush on his best friend George. She wants to be understanding and asks for help. The nurse should explain that:
   a. Sexual identity is usually set by the beginning of adolescence so Mike is gay and it is good she is prepared to accept this.
   b. She should show Mike that a gay lifestyle is unacceptable to her so that he will choose not to assume this lifestyle to prevent rejection from his family.
   c. For many adolescents, a same-sex crush may reflect a temporary, experimental stage in which questioning of sexual preference may occur but does not affect later heterosexuality.
   d. Gays and lesbians realize their sexual orientation during early childhood so these feelings are likely meaningless if Mike has not shown a sexual preference for men prior to this time.

2. Ms. Parker also expresses concern that Mike has been alternating from a rebellious, very independent child to a very playful and silly young man who needs family guidance. She fears he may have mental problems. You would explain that:
   a. Mike may have a split personality and should be committed to a mental institution.
   b. Young adolescents often fluctuate between testing independence and wanting parental approval.
   c. Mike shows signs of regression and needs to have psychological counseling to help him to control his spiritedness.
   d. If Mike begins to show moodiness and seclusion he will need constant supervision to prevent his spending time reflecting on himself.

3. During late adolescence which of the following behaviors would be cause for concern?
   a. The teen enters the work force or joins the military after finishing school.
   b. A young woman or man dates a variety of individuals.
   c. The teen chooses friends who are 10 years older and wiser about the world than the teen is.
   d. Parents of the adolescent encourage the adolescent to use the home as a base for friendships and personal activities.

4. Which of the following indicates the area of concern for adolescents with the topic area?
   a. Food and eating habits are a concern because gaining 2 or 3 pounds can make adolescent girls depressed and because anorexia and bulimia may emerge during these years.
   b. Peer pressure is natural; families who attempt to model safe habits and practices could confuse the teen.
   c. Sex education should be provided to adolescents by peers and older adolescents to prevent rejection of the information by the teen.
   d. Risk-taking behavior is always a result of the teen's lack of knowledge of the consequences of the risky actions so peer teaching must be done to ensure proper behavior.

12

Early and Middle Adulthood

CHAPTER OVERVIEW

Chapter 12 discusses growth and development in early and late adulthood. An overview of adult growth and development theories is provided.

✪ Be sure to review the Learning Objectives from the text.

✦ Be sure to FIRST perform Improving Concentration exercises described in the Introduction before proceeding with the next exercise.

Part 1

Indicate the order in which you find the following major headings in this chapter.

_____ Development in Middle Adulthood

_____ Adult Growth and Development Theories

_____ Development in Early Adulthood

Part 2

Complete the following statements related to the major headings and key points.

1. Development continues throughout life and during

adulthood; periods of _____ alternate with periods of _____ .

2. The two subheadings found in this chapter under "Development in Early Adulthood" contain the age ranges of _____ to _____ years, and _____ to _____ years.

3. Adults must meet certain _____ _____ to mature comfortably.

Part 3 Key Terms: Knowledge Check

Unscramble the letters to identify the term that best matches the definition.

1. yevantigiret _____
   Middle adults decide to pass on learning and share skills with younger generations

2. manicity _____
   Individuals choose to establish relationships with others

3. asilotoin _____ _____
   Individuals choose to remain detached from others

4. ilemfid anitornist _____ _____
   Can involve a sense of failure in the chosen profession, feelings of sexual inadequacy, fear of inevitable death, or frustration with aging parents or grown children

Part 4

Indicate if the following tasks or the psychosocial development is associated with early adulthood (E) or middle adulthood (M).

1. _____ The individual assists children to become responsible adults.

2. _____ A focus is on strengthening the relationship with his or her partner.

3. _____ The individual becomes involved with civic and religious group activities.

4. _____ The individual must deal with and assist aging parents.

5. _____ A necessary accomplishment is choosing a relationship style.

6. ____ Intimacy versus isolation is the challenge for this developmental age.

7. ____ The virtues that must be developed include production, caring, and cooperation.

8. ____ Generativity versus self-absorption is the challenge for this group.

Column II

a. Early adult transition

b. Catch thirties

c. Payoff years

d. Settling down

e. Time of renewal

Part 5

Match the concepts and definitions in column I with the period or phase of development in column II.

Column I

1. ____ Occurs between ages 45 and 65; Levinson indicates the transitions include the balance of choices.

2. ____ Sheehy's phase of adulthood in which the individual establishes a new home and focuses on career goals

3. ____ Occurs during the forties and fifties; there is a changing self-image and the individual must face own mortality.

4. ____ The time between age 18 and 22 when the person must establish an adult identity and establish personal goals.

5. ____ A time from 33 to 39 years of age when the major transitions include a balance of choices.

Part 6 Short Answer Exercises

Complete the following fill-in-the-blank and short answer questions.

1. Individual _____ and _____ are more influential than chronological age in determining patterns of development.

2. Briefly discuss three of the stages an adult goes through between the ages of 20 to 30 years. _____

3. List three stages an adult goes through between the ages of 30 to 40 years. _____

4. List the activities that an individual may undertake during middle adulthood. _____

13

Older Adulthood and Aging

CHAPTER OVERVIEW

Chapter 13 discusses the development of the older adult and concepts of aging. Developmental theories are addressed, and an overview of demographics and population trends is provided.

✪ Be sure to review the Learning Objectives from the text.

✍ Be sure to FIRST perform Improving Concentration exercises described in the Introduction before proceeding with the next exercise.

Part 1

Complete the following statements related to the major headings and key points of the chapter.

1. List the theorists discussed under the major heading "Developmental Theories of Older Adulthood"

   _____, _____,
   _____, and _____.

2. The final major heading in this chapter is _____ and _____

   _____.

3. The process of aging is a _____ of earlier development.

4. _____, _____, and _____ are significant concerns for older adults.

5. Society must examine _____ concerns related to the expanding older population.

Part 2 Key Terms: Knowledge Check

Review the key terms in the chapter. Unscramble the term in column I and indicate the letter of the correct definition in column II.

Column I

1. _____ (tolymatir)

2. _____ (gisame)

3. _____ (togyrolegon)

Column II

a. Labeling and discriminating against individuals as they grow older

b. The study of the aging process in all its dimensions (physical, psychological, economic, sociologic, and spiritual)

c. A term for death; reflected on by the older adults, particularly after the death of a spouse

Part 3

Associate the theorist with the following statements on the development of older adults by indicating H for Havighurst, E for Erikson, L for Levinson, and S for Sheehy.

1. _____ The challenge of this age is ego integrity versus despair.

2. _____ Older adulthood involves the task of adjusting to the death of a spouse or companion.

3. _____ A task of the older adult is to establish social relationships with persons of same age and with younger persons.

4. _____ Older adults need to feel comfortable with the changes that occur and to attain the dignity that is part of aging.

5. _____ Necessary accomplishments in older adulthood include the need to balance choices and achieve stability, and accept life choices.

6. _____ Life after age 65 is a time for adults to find a new balance of involvement with society and with the self.

7. _____ Successful transition in older adulthood results in wisdom and stability.

8. _____ Renunciation, wisdom, and dignity are virtues the older adult should develop.

Part 4

Indicate if the following actions by a nurse would be appropriate (A) or inappropriate (I) as discussed in this chapter.

1. _____ The nurse explains to an older adult that the changes related to aging are pathologic and cannot be adapted to so acceptance of pending disability is important.

2. _____ Care to an older adult in the hospital is adjusted, when possible, to allow the client to watch her morning gospel show as she does every morning at home.

3. _____ Avoid discussing the death of the client's spouse or peers, or past activities, to prevent morbid thinking or depression.

4. _____ Expect that clients who are older will be more concerned about the opinion of others and will respond to stress more violently because of their age.

5. _____ Limit research in nursing to persons aged 65 to 75 because this group is the fastest growing segment of the population of the United States.

6. _____ Assist family members to arrange for home assistance for an aging parent to help the

parent live at home and retain independence as long as possible.

7. _____ Encourage older adults to choose and plan activities before and after retirement because activity is necessary for life.

8. _____ Discuss exciting trips the older adult should take because their finances are better at this time than during their earlier years and they can afford to enjoy life.

Part 5

Complete the following fill-in-the blank questions.

1. Financially, most people (older adults) have to adjust to a _____ _____ after retirement.

2. People with fixed habits and attitudes may face _____ adjusting to change.

3. Participation in _____ work is rewarding for many older individuals: being a guide at a zoo or helping babies and children, or delivering meals to the homebound.

4. Although spirituality and religion are often thought of as _____, they are not necessarily the _____ thing.

5. Life expectancy continues to _____ in the United States and Canada.

14

Death and Dying

CHAPTER OVERVIEW

Chapter 14 discusses death and dying and its relationship to growth and development. The stages of dying are addressed, as well as the influences of culture, ethnicity, spirituality, and religion on the death experience. The impact of death on the family is discussed.

✪ Be sure to review the Learning Objectives from the text.

✤ Be sure to FIRST perform Improving Concentration exercises described in the Introduction before proceeding with the next exercise.

Part 1

Indicate the order in which you find the following major headings in this chapter.

_____ Influences of Culture, Ethnicity, and Religion

_____ Death's Impact on the Family

_____ Spirituality and Death

_____ Stages of Dying

Part 2

Complete the following statements.

1. Death is a _____ part of the total life process.

2. Families who face the impending death of a member may endure enormous _____. They need encouragement to _____ their _____.

3. Most people, if they do not die suddenly, pass through definite _____ during the dying process. The ultimate goal is _____.

Part 3 Key Terms: Knowledge Check

Review the key terms in the chapter. Unscramble the letters to reveal the term or terms that best match(es) the definition.

1. _____ _____ (etircave spesedrino)
The individual concentrates on past losses; a verbal stage of grief

2. _____ (thecetmand)
When an individual gradually separates from the world so a two-way communication no longer exists with people around him or her; the final stage of dying

3. _____ _____ (ritalnem sleslin)
A state in which an individual faces a medical condition that will end in death within a limited period

4. _____ _____ (etrarpropay poiserndes)
A nonverbal stage of grief in which a person who is dying realizes the impact of loss

Part 4

Answer these statements true (T) or false (F).

1. _____ A family with a member who is dying may experience stress more keenly than the person does.

2. _____ Everyday problems such as babysitting and transportation are seldom of concern to the family when the death of member occurs because neighbors will help.

3. _____ Adults should not address death with a child because children will not be able to comprehend it and will suffer nightmares if exposed to the concept of dying.

4. _____ The most important developmental task of older adulthood is to delay death as long as possible.

5. _____ Spiritual support may take the form of compassionate care and acceptance of personal beliefs.

Part 5

Match the suggestion for helping a person cope with death, found in column I, with the stage of dealing with death, found in column II, and the statements found in column III.

Column I

1. _____ Provide physical care, be there, keep the room lighted.

2. _____ Continue to include person in conversation.

3. _____ Try to assist in client's wishes; offer spiritual assistance.

4. _____ Answer questions honestly, do not argue.

5. _____ Listen, do not take the client's behavior personally.

6. _____ Offer encouragement, allow person to rest.

Column II

a. Anger

b. Depression

c. Denial

d. Detachment

e. Acceptance

f. Bargaining

Column III

g. "No, not me"

h. "Why me?"

i. "Yes me"

j. "My time is close, and it's OK"

k. "Yes me, but . . ., If I could just live until"

l. No communication

Part 6 Short Answer Exercises

Complete the following short answer questions.

1. What are the three levels of spiritual support mentioned by Bernard and Schneider (1996)?

_____

_____

2. Discuss how culturally death may be viewed in opposite ways; focus on public versus private and grieving versus joy.

_____

3. What are the key characteristics for each stage of dying; example: for Anger—rage is key.

_____

15

Organization of the Human Body

Common Acronyms or Terms

DNA	MASH
H_2O	RBC
LLQ	RLQ
LUQ	RUQ
m	WBC

CHAPTER OVERVIEW

Chapter 15 presents the human body as a precisely structured arrangement of liquids, gases, and solids. It summarizes medical terminology, chemistry, and basic information about anatomy and physiology.

✪ Be sure to review the Learning Objectives from the text.

✔ Be sure to FIRST perform Improving Concentration exercises described in the Introduction before proceeding with the next exercise.

Part 1 Matching

Choose one of the sections from the topic outline to correctly define where this information can be found.

1. _____ The difference between chemical and physical changes

2. _____ Examples of suffixes can be found in this section.

3. _____ The difference between meiosis and mitosis

4. _____ The basis organization of elements and compounds

5. _____ The anatomic terms that apply to cavities and quadrants

a. Chemistry and Life

b. Medical Terminology

c. Structural Levels in the Body

d. Body Directions

Part 2 Key Terms: Knowledge Check

Below is a list of definitions. Choose from the list of key terms found in the beginning of the chapter, note the words you indicated you did not know, and write each word beside the correct definition. The number in parenthesis indicates the number of letters in the correct word.

Smallest part of any element (4) _____

Basic unit of structure and formation for all living things (4) _____

Formed from chromosomes, they carry specific information about inherited characteristics (4) _____

Fine, hairlike extensions (5) _____

A group of different types of tissues forming in a specific way to perform a definite function (5) _____

Imaginary flat surface that divides the human body into sections (5) _____

Posterior, back cavity (6) _____

Complex protein structures that speed up chemical reactions (6) _____

Medical terms based on the names of people (6) _____

Vertical division of the body longitudinally into front and back parts (6) _____

Group of organs (6) _____

Cells of the same type and structure that have a specific function (6) _____

Words formed by combining letters of a word or phrase (7) _____

Study of body structure (7) _____

A pure, simple chemical (7) _____

Cell division producing eggs or sperm that contain one-half of chromosomes (7) _____

Anterior, front cavity (7) _____

Blend of two or more substances that mix together to form a compound (7) _____

Process in which cells divide to reproduce exact genetic duplicates (7) _____

Center (of an atom) (7) _____

Substance formed when atoms of two or more elements react chemically (8) _____

Surrounds the outer boundary of the cell and is capable of selective chemical permeability (8) _____

Division into four parts using horizontal and vertical lines (8) _____

Vertical division of the body into right and left sides (8) _____

Cell area not located in the nucleus (9) _____

Large muscle that separates ventral cavities (9) _____

Horizontal division of the body into upper and lower parts (10) _____

DNA that is located mostly in the nucleus—forms genes (10) _____

Collectively, all parts that make up a cell (10) _____

Study of how the body functions (10) _____

Ability to process, obtain energy from and create new products using the chemicals found in foods (10) _____

The dynamic balance of anatomy and physiology (11) _____

Part 3

Complete the paragraph by filling in the space with the correct term.

1. Matter occupies _____ and has weight. Element, compound and _____ are the three _____ of matter. Solid, _____, and gas are the three _____ of matter.

2. The physical and emotional equilibrium a person strives to maintain is known as _____.

Chemistry is the basis for the dynamic balance of _____ and physiology.

Part 4 True or False

Answer these statements true (T) or false (F).

1. _____ Water is capable of undergoing both physical and chemical change.

2. _____ Connective tissue lines the hollow portions of blood vessels.

3. _____ Systems are made up of cells.

4. _____ Physical change occurs when outward and chemical properties change.

5. _____ All medical terms have a prefix.

6. _____ Cytology is the science of the study of cells.

Part 5

Choose from the list of numbers below to correctly complete the following sentences.

1. All matter can be broken down into _____ different elements.

2. As many as _____ cells can fit on the head of a pin.

3. Water forms when _____ hydrogen atoms combine with _____ oxygen atoms.

4. Elements compose approximately _____% of human weight.

5. DNA builds the protein the body needs from endless combinations of these _____ amino acids.

6. The human body is approximately _____% water.

7. There are _____ kinds of matter that exist in _____ states.

7

111

20

1

60

3

1,000

99

2

Part 6

Examples of different tissues are listed below. Place the number of the tissue type in column I beside the correct tissue listed listed in column II.

Column I

1. Epithelial

2. Connective

3. Muscle

4. Nerve

Column II

a. _____ Blood

b. _____ Neurons

c. _____ Calluses

d. _____ Bone

e. _____ Cardiac

f. _____ Glands

g. _____ Adipose

h. _____ Skeletal

Part 7

Now complete the puzzle filling in one letter for each block, until all the words have been used and all the blocks in the puzzle have been filled.

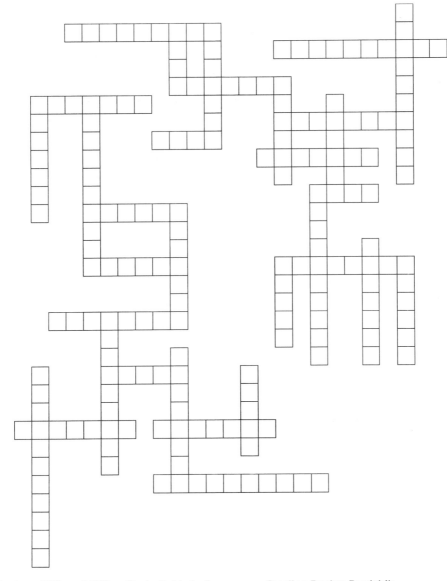

16

The Integumentary System

Common Acronyms or Terms

UV

CHAPTER OVERVIEW

Chapter 16 states the components of the integumentary system; the skin and its accessory organs and outlines its primary functions; protection, metabolism, thermoregulation, sensation, and communication.

✪ Be sure to review the Learning Objectives from the text.

✔ Be sure to FIRST perform Improving Concentration exercises described in the Introduction before proceeding with the next exercise.

Part 1

Complete the names of the following subheadings found in the chapter.

1. S_ _ _
2. A_ _ _ _ _ _ _ _ S_ _ _ _ _ _ _ _ _
3. T_ _ _ _ _ _ _ _ _ _ _ _ _ _ _
4. S_ _ _ _ _ _ A_ _ _ _ _ _ _ _

Part 2

Complete the sentence with the appropriate word from the key terms.

1. Liver or age spots are clusters of melanin that are similar to _____.
2. The corium is also known as the _____.
3. Integument literally means _____.
4. The medical term for excessive perspiration is _____.
5. These are a specialized type of sudoriferous glands that secrete milk. _____
6. Maintenance of the internal temperature of the body occurs through a process called _____.

Part 3 True or False

Answer these statements true (T) or false (F).

1. _____ Living in a nursing home setting combined with a decrease in milk or calcium intake can double the risk of vitamin D deficiency.
2. _____ Freckles are a result of melanocytes that do not make enough melanin.
3. _____ Sebaceous glands can also be called oil glands.
4. _____ Gray hair results when there is a total loss of melanin to the hair shaft.
5. _____ Older people tend to show an increase in skin turgor.

Part 4

Fill in the space with the correct term.

1. Damage to the base layer of the epithelium takes longer to heal because the damaged skin has lost its _____ (reproductive) structures.
2. _____ and vitamin deficiencies can cause skin and hair to be dull, _____, and flaky.

3. Water loss through _____ causes a cooling effect.

4. This type of connective tissue has a root word that means "glue." _____

5. _____ tissue is the layer beneath the dermis and on top of the layer of muscle.

Part 5 Multiple Choice

Circle the letter corresponding to the correct answer.

1. The medical term for hair loss is:
   a. Vitiligo
   b. Desquamation
   c. Alopecia
   d. Corium
2. The transfer of heat from a surface to a surrounding gas is known as:
   a. Evaporation
   b. Convection
   c. Conduction
   d. Radiation
3. Diaphoresis is associated with glands called:
   a. Sudoriferous
   b. Sebaceous
   c. Subcutaneous
   d. Squamous
4. A pigment found in red blood cells is:
   a. Ceruminal
   b. Carotene
   c. Sebum
   d. Hemoglobin
5. The yellowish pigment that is a precursor to vitamin A is:
   a. Collagen
   b. Keratin
   c. Carotene
   d. Melanin

Part 6

Please read the clinical information and make the BEST choice based only on the information you are given.

You admit Mrs. Thurman, a 90-pound, 78-year-old widow, to bed 201B and as you are taking her history you notice that she is shivering. You recognize that:
a. Shivering is a way the body attempts to regulate temperature in the adult.
b. She is at risk for dehydration due to diaphoresis and evaporation.
c. Older people often have difficulty keeping warm.
d. Obtaining an accurate admission temperature will be important.
   1. a and d
   2. a, b, c, and d
   3. a, b, and d
   4. a, c, and d

17

✪ Be sure to review the Learning Objectives from the text.

✔ Be sure to FIRST perform Improving Concentration exercises described in the Introduction before proceeding with the next exercise.

Fluid and Electrolyte Balance

Part 1

Indicate the order in which the following major headings appear in the chapter.

_____ Fluid and Electrolyte Transport

_____ Effects of Aging on the System

_____ Fluid and Electrolyte Balance

_____ Body Fluids

_____ Acid–Base Balance

_____ Homeostasis

Common Acronyms or Terms

ADH	IVF
ANP	KCL
ATP	mEq
CO_2	mL
CSF	mL/d
ECF	NaCL
HCL	O_2
ICF	pH

Part 2 Key Terms: Knowledge Check
Opposites Attract/Matching Terms

Choose a term from column I that is the opposite of a term from column II.

Column I

Hypertonic	_____
Acid	_____
Anion	_____
Extracellular	_____

Column II

Base

Intracellular

Hypotonic

Cation

CHAPTER OVERVIEW

Chapter 17 reviews the role of water and electrolytes in the maintenance of homeostasis as well as the systems of fluid transport that are involved.

Part 3 Something in Common

Draw line from the item in column I to the item in column II with which it has the strongest connection.

Column I

Osmosis   _____

Electrolyte   _____

Isotonic   _____

Solute   _____

Edema   _____

Column II

Salt

Interstitial

Diffusion

Ion

Homeostasis

Part 4

Complete the sentence with the correct term.

1. Intracellular literally means _____ the cell.

2. The mechanisms by which the body enhances or intensifies the original stimulus is known as _____ _____.

3. The suffix meaning "stopping or controlling" combined with the root word meaning "constant or sameness," which describes the dynamic process through which the body maintains balance, is called _____.

4. _____ is the medical term for severe, generalized edema.

5. A transfer that can occur without energy is known as _____ _____.

6. The ability of a membrane to allow molecules to pass through it is known as _____.

Part 5 Multiple Choice

Circle the letter corresponding to the correct answer.

1. A chemical system set up to resist changes particularly in the level of pH is a:
   a. Base
   b. Acid
   c. Buffer
   d. Salt

2. Dehydration results from the excessive loss of:
   a. H_2O_2
   b. H^+
   c. OH
   d. H_2O

3. Filtration requires:
   a. Sodium and potassium pump
   b. Diffusion
   c. Osmosis
   d. Mechanical pressure

18

The Musculoskeletal System

Common Acronyms or Terms

ROM

CHAPTER OVERVIEW

Chapter 18 discusses the various components of the body system that works together to enable physical movement.

❂ Be sure to review the Learning Objectives from the text.

✔ Be sure to FIRST perform Improving Concentration exercises described in the Introduction before proceeding with the next exercise.

Part 1

Indicate the order in which these subheadings are found in the chapter.

_____ The Skeleton

_____ Muscle Contractions

_____ The Muscles

_____ Formation of Bone Tissue

_____ Divisions of the Skeleton

Part 2

Match the definitions in column I with the terms in column II.

Column I

1. _____ Synovial joints that are freely movable in various directions

2. _____ Portion of the skeleton containing the bones of the extremities and appendages of the body

3. _____ Cardiac muscle—the middle muscle layer of the heart

4. _____ Muscles that control involuntary motion inside body organs

5. _____ Medical term for a dent or depression

6. _____ Ability of a muscle to stretch

7. _____ Term for forward movement

8. _____ Single muscle or group of muscles that initiate movement

9. _____ Hole through which blood vessels, ligaments, and nerves pass

10. _____ Term for backward movement

11. _____ Moving away form the midline of the body

12. _____ Large process located on the femur (for example)

13. _____ Bending the foot so that the bones are pointed downward

14. _____ Small horseshoe-shaped bone below the mandible and above the larynx

15. _____ Ability to respond to a stimulus

Column II

a. Extensibility

b. Trochanter

c. Protraction

d. Abduction

e. Foramen

f. Hyoid

g. Diarthrosis

h. Plantar flexion

i. Irritability

j. Prime mover

k. Fossa

l. Myocardium

m. Smooth

n. Appendicular

o. Retraction

Part 3

Determine whether the term listed below involves structure (anatomy) or function (physiology), indicating with an S or F.

1. _____ Masseter

2. _____ Joints

3. _____ Osteoclasts

4. _____ Xiphoid process

5. _____ ATP

6. _____ Manubrium

7. _____ Acetabulum

8. _____ Hormones

Part 4 Critical Thinking

1. Discuss how the normal changes associated with the aging process can affect the gait of older adults and make them more vulnerable to falling.

   _____

   _____

2. List two voluntary, involuntary, and protective functions of muscles.

   _____

   _____

   _____

Part 5 The Numbers Game

Choose from the list of numbers below to correctly complete the following sentences. Some numbers may be used more than once.

1. More than _____% of the total bones in the human body are found in the hands and wrists.

2. Skeletal muscle comprises _____% of total body weight.

3. Each muscle fiber is about the size of a human hair and can hold about _____ times its own weight.

4. The angle of the pelvic opening is less than _____% in men and greater than _____% in women.

5. The skull is made up of _____ bones.

6. There are _____ thoracic vertebrae.

0

40

1,000

90

28

12

25

Part 6 Clinical Situation

Mr. Quasimoto was admitted to your unit before undergoing a battery of surgeries to correct a combination of congenital defects. On admission you note that he is cross-eyed, a hunchback, and has his head permanently drawn to one side. The medical terms for these three conditions are _____.

Part 7 Multiple Choice

Circle the letter corresponding to the correct answer.

1. The intercostal muscles are located:
   a. Between the shoulder blades
   b. Between the ribs
   c. Between the clavicles
   d. Between the vertebrae

2. Hard, fibrous connective tissue that covers most of the outside of the bone is called:
   a. Periosteum
   b. Bursae
   c. Marrow
   d. Cartilage

3. The cervical vertebrae are located in the:
   a. Sacrum
   b. Sternum
   c. Thorax
   d. Neck

Part 8 Puzzle Parts

Below is a list of definitions. Choose one word from the list of key terms at the beginning of the chapter and write that word beside the definition. The number in parentheses tells you the number of letters in the correct word. Following the four sets of definitions are four puzzles to be completed, with one letter for each block in the puzzle until all the blocks have been filled.

Puzzle 1 Definitions

1. _____ Upper bone of leg—supports weight of upper body, thigh bone (5)

2. _____ Weight-bearing long bone of the lower leg (5)

3. _____ Non–weight-bearing bone attached to the tibia at the upper end (6)

4. _____ In the fetus this bone is three separate bones, the ilium, ischium, and pubis (6)

5. _____ Five parts in children, one solid bone in adults; anchors the pelvis (6)

6. _____ Kneecap (7)

Puzzle 2 Definitions

1. _____ Larger, forearm bone with two hollows in its upper end (4)

2. _____ Eight wrist bones that support the base of the palm (6)

3. _____ Smaller forearm bone, lies beside the ulna (6)

4. _____ Single, long bone found in upper arm (7)

Puzzle 3 Definitions

1. _____ Cavity formed by the ribs (6)

2. _____ Front boundary of upper part of thorax (7)

3. _____ Function to provide body movement, blood circulation, and heat production (7)

4. _____ Opposite the clavicles on each side of the back (7)

5. _____ Two thin long bones attached to the sternum (8)

Puzzle 4 Definitions

1. _____ Term that describes the place at which bones attach to each other (5)

2. _____ Sacs filled with synovial fluid that ease movement and reduce friction (6)

3. _____ This substance when red is responsible for hematopoiesis; when yellow is mostly fat (6)

4. _____ These tough cords attach muscle to bones (7)

5. _____ Connective tissue organized into fibers; functions as a shock absorber (9)

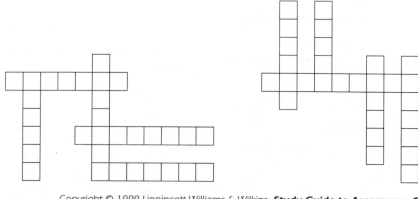

19

The Nervous System

Common Acronyms or Terms

ANS

CNS

CSF

EEG

kg

PNS

CHAPTER OVERVIEW

Chapter 19 presents the nervous system as the overall director of body systems. It explores its role in communicating messages from one system to another as well as processing information from the outside environment and storing information for future reference.

✪ Be sure to review the Learning Objectives from the text.

✔ Be sure to FIRST perform Improving Concentration exercises described in the Introduction before proceeding with the next exercise.

Part 1

Complete the subheadings under the following major headings.

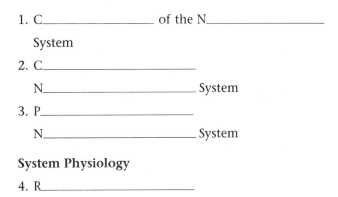

Structure and Function

1. C_____ of the N_____
   System

2. C_____
   N_____ System

3. P_____
   N_____ System

System Physiology

4. R_____

Part 2

Choose from the list of key terms to find the one that describes each definition listed below.

1. The "circle" of nerve fibers in the reflex center of the spinal cord that sends and receives messages.

   _____

2. Neurons that serve to integrate signals between the neurons of various parts of the CNS.

   _____

3. This part of the cerebral cortex controls sensations of touch and spatial ability.

   _____

4. A chemical that an axon releases to allow nerve impulses to cross the synapse and reach the dendrites.

   _____

5. A band of 200 million neurons connecting the right and left hemispheres.

   _____

6. The organized, rapid exchange of sodium and potassium ions across a cell membrane, which spreads like an electric current.

   _____

7. The part of the limbic system that functions in learning and long-term memory.

   _____

8. An automatic or involuntary response to a stimulus.

   _____

9. A lymph like fluid that forms a protective cushion around and within the CNS.

10. Crossing of the nerve tracts within the brain's medulla.

_____

11. End organs that initially receive stimuli from outside and within the body. They are usually classified in three ways.

_____

12. Fatty covering surrounding the axon.

_____

13. They outnumber neurons five to one and support and connect nervous tissue, but do not transmit impulses.

_____

14. Second largest part functions in movement.

_____

15. This portion of the nervous system is divided into sympathetic and parasympathetic.

_____

Part 3 Matched Pairs

The terms in column I are related to another term in column II. Draw a line from one related term to the other.

Column I

Sensory   _____

Cranial nerve VII   _____

Parasympathetic   _____

Cranial nerve II   _____

Motor   _____

Study of nervous system   _____

Cranial nerve X   _____

Sympathetic   _____

Plexus   _____

Brain and spinal cord   _____

Neurotransmitter   _____

Pons   _____

Column II

Optic

Vagus

Neurology

Acetylcholine

Afferent

Group of spinal nerves

Homeostasis

Facial

Bridge

Efferent

Emergency

Central nervous system

Part 4

Complete the sentence.

1. The thalamus is responsible for _____ and strong emotions.

2. The brain is covered with three meninges; dura mater, _____, and pia mater.

3. A neuron consists of a cell body, axon, and _____.

4. The part of the brain responsible for muscle control is the _____.

5. The portion of the brain stem responsible for vital body functions, such as heart rate, is the _____.

6. Primary functions of the nervous system are _____ and control.

7. The _____ lobe of the cerebrum is responsible for vision.

8. The _____ regulates body functions such as the sleep–wake cycle.

9. The spinal cord serves as a reflex center and conducts impulses to and from the _____.

Part 5

Each sentence below is accurate EXCEPT for one word. Change one word in each sentence to make it true.

1. The neuron is the basic structural and functional organ of the nervous system.

2. Axons carry impulses toward the cell body.

3. People who have had a cerebrovascular accident (stroke) affecting one brain hemisphere exhibit symptoms (paralysis) on the same side of the body.

4. An action potential takes only seconds.

5. Peristalsis is an example of voluntary control.

6. The "all or none" law describes how impulses can be partially transmitted.

7. The temporal lobe is responsible for higher mental processes.

8. Generally, nerve cells can reproduce themselves.

9. The cerebral cortex is the innermost part of the brain.

10. The dura mater lies closely over the brain and spinal cord. It is thin and vascular.

20

The Endocrine System

Common Acronyms or Terms

ACTH	LH
ADH	MIH
ANP	MSH
CRH	PIH
FSH	PRH
GH	PRL
GHIH	PTH
GNRH	TSH
GRH, GHRH	TRH
HCG	T_3
ICSH	T_4

CHAPTER OVERVIEW

Chapter 20 discusses the function of glands and hormones in the maintenance of body functions.

✪ Be sure to review the Learning Objectives from the text.

✔ Be sure to FIRST perform Improving Concentration exercises described in the Introduction before proceeding with the next exercise.

Part 1

Complete the following subheadings found under the major headings.

Structure and Functions

1. T_____ Gland

2. P_____

3. P_____ Glands

System Physiology

4. S_____

   R_____

5. N_____

   F_____

Part 2 Multiple Choice

Circle the letter corresponding to the correct answer.

1. The parathyroids regulate the amount of:
   a. Potassium and chloride
   b. Calcium and phosphorus
   c. Sodium and potassium
   d. Potassium and calcium

2. The nervous system tissue of the hypothalamus controls the:
   a. Parathyroid gland
   b. Pineal gland
   c. Pituitary gland
   d. Thymus gland

3. Mechanisms that influence hormonal blood levels include:
   a. "All or none" principle
   b. Positive feedback
   c. Action potential
   d. Negative feedback

4. The gland responsible for controlling the body's rate of metabolism is the:
   a. Parathyroid
   b. Thyroid
   c. Thymus
   d. Pancreas

5. This gland secretes hormones that play a role in cellular immunity:
   a. Thymus
   b. Thyroid
   c. Parathyroid
   d. Pineal

Part 3

Choose the number of the gland that secretes the hormones listed below.

1. Adrenals
2. Thyroid
3. Pancreas
4. Pituitary

a. _____ Growth hormone
b. _____ Insulin
c. _____ Catecholamines
d. _____ Calcitonin
e. _____ Oxytocin
f. _____ Glucocorticoids
g. _____ Thyroid-stimulating hormone
h. _____ Glucagon
i. _____ Vasopressin

Part 4 Riddle Me This

Complete the statements by filling in the blanks.

1. I am a gland the size of a small, green vegetable, located in a hollow called the sella turcica. I am the _____ gland.
2. I am the largest of the endocrine glands with a wing on each side of the throat. I am the _____ gland.
3. I am a tiny structure found at the top of the third ventricle. I am shaped like a cone and I am called the _____ gland.
4. I sit like a hat on top of a kidney. I am the _____ gland.
5. I am both an endocrine and an exocrine gland. I am located behind the stomach. I am the _____.

Part 5 True or False

Indicate in the blank provided if the statement is true or false. Correct the false statements.

1. Renin is a hormone that is produced by the juxta-glomerular apparatus that assists in the control of blood pressure. _____
2. Prostaglandins are hormones whose effects are localized to the area in which they are produced. _____
3. It is possible for an organ, under certain conditions, to temporarily be an endocrine gland. _____
4. Epinephrine and norepinephrine are made from amino acids and are secreted by the adrenal medulla. _____
5. Erythropoietin, a glycoprotein that stimulates red blood cell production, is produced in the liver of adults. _____

Part 6 Double Take

Complete the statement by filling in the blank.

1. Gl_____ acts opposite insulin, raising blood sugar.
2. Pi_____ produces melatonin.
3. Ad_____ is the anterior lobe of the pituitary.
4. Th_____ stimulates the production of T lymphocytes.
5. Pi_____ is the hypophysis, the anterior lobe of the pituitary.
6. Th_____ secretes thyroxine and triiodothyronine.
7. Ad_____ are the suprarenal glands.
8. Gl_____ is stored sugar, which breaks down into glucose.

Part 7 True or False

Answer the statements true (T) or false (F). Correct the false statements.

1. _____ Hydrocortisone is a corticosteroid.

2. _____ The parathyroids are small, nonessential glands.

3. _____ The exocrine portion of the pancreas contains the islets of Langerhans.

4. _____ Prostaglandins are specialized amino acids that were first isolated in the seminal fluid of the prostrate.

5. _____ The neurohypophysis of the pituitary gland releases oxytocin and vasopressin.

6. _____ Hormones are chemical regulators that integrate and coordinate body activities.

7. _____ The hypothalamus is a large, simple portion of the brain attached to the pituitary.

8. _____ Beta cells of the pancreas secrete insulin.

9. _____ Endocrine glands secrete hormones directly into the bloodstream.

10. _____ The endocrine and circulatory systems operate independently of each other.

21

The Sensory System

CHAPTER OVERVIEW

Chapter 21 presents an overview of the sensory system and describes how it functions to provide protection and mechanisms for experiencing the world by detecting environmental changes.

✪ Be sure to review the Learning Objectives from the text.

✍ Be sure to FIRST perform Improving Concentration exercises described in the Introduction before proceeding with the next exercise.

Part 1

Identify if the following subheadings are found under the major headings: **a. Structure and Function, b. System Physiology, or c. Effects of Aging on the System.**

1. _____ The Ear

2. _____ Balance and Equilibrium

3. _____ Smell

4. _____ Eye and Vision Changes

5. _____ Other Sensations

Part 2

Supply the correct answer to the definitions listed below.

1. _____
   Waxy substance secreted by the lining of the auditory canal

2. _____
   Adjustment by the lens to make a sharp, clear image

3. _____
   Produce tears and is located at the lateral canthus

4. _____
   Collective name of the malleus, the incus, and the stapes

5. _____
   Transparent, gelatin-like material located behind the lens

6. _____
   Located inside the temporal bone, this structure is snail shaped.

7. _____
   Located in muscles, tendons and joints, indicate body position

8. _____
   Specialized neurons of the eye, useful in night vision

9. _____
   Nearsightedness

10. _____
    Point where the optic nerve meets the retina

Part 3 The Name Game

Answer these questions in the spaces provided.

1. List the five senses and at least one organ associated with each.

   _____

2. Name two cranial nerves involved in ocular functioning.

   _____

3. Name the portion of the inner ear responsible for balance.

   _____

4. Name three of the six extraocular muscles that control eye movements.

_____

5. Name the portion of the ear responsible for the transmission of sound.

_____

Part 4 Clinical Thinking

You are performing the initial home health assessment for 78-year-old Ernest Jackson. He tells you that he has noticed that when he reads he has to hold the paper at arms' length or the letters are blurry and that he has noticed a steady decline in his hearing. You document the clinical terms for the these sensory changes as:

1. _____
2. _____

Part 5

Change one word to make the sentence correct.

1. Proprioceptors in the mouth provide information about taste.

2. Cones are useful in night vision.

3. The temporal lobe of the brain interprets visual images.

4. The eustachian tube closes during swallowing or yawning.

5. Cranial nerve I is the oculomotor nerve.

Part 6 Multiple Choice

Circle the letter corresponding to the correct answer.

1. The pinna, or external ear, is also known as the:
   a. Ossicle
   b. Auricle
   c. Abducens
   d. Incus

2. The organ of Corti is located inside the:
   a. Stapes
   b. Malleus
   c. Cochlea
   d. Auricle

3. The clinical term that describes a sensation that the room is spinning is called:
   a. Vertigo
   b. Presbycusis
   c. Tympanitis
   d. Tinnitus

4. The "white of the eye" is also known as the:
   a. Cornea
   b. Retina
   c. Iris
   d. Sclera

22

The Cardiovascular System

Common Acronyms or Terms

AV

BP

CO

HR

LAD

LCA

LCX

LMCA

RAC

SA

SV

SVR

CHAPTER OVERVIEW

Chapter 22 describes the role of the heart and blood vessels in the delivery of nutrients and the removal of waste products from the human body.

✪ Be sure to review the Learning Objectives from the text.

✔ Be sure to FIRST perform Improving Concentration exercises described in the Introduction before proceeding with the next exercise.

Part 1

Complete the words or phrases that indicate the name of major headings or subheadings.

1. S_____

   P_____

2. C_____

   C_____

3. Effects of A_____ on the S_____

4. B_____

   V_____

5. C_____

   O_____

Part 2

Choose from the list below the word or term that best matches the numbered word or term.

1. _____ Cardiac output

2. _____ First heart sound

3. _____ Arteries

4. _____ Left coronary artery

5. _____ Pacemaker

6. _____ Hepatic artery

7. _____ Second heart sound

8. _____ Bicuspid

9. _____ Preload

10. _____ "Receiving station"

a. Mitral

b. SA node

c. Ventricles relax

d. "Stretching force"

e. AV node

f. Branches off abdominal aorta

g. Stroke volume × heart rate

h. Resistance vessels

i. Ventricles contract

j. Branches off ascending aorta

Part 3 Correct Quartets

Choose the correct word or prefix to complete the definitions from the list of key terms.

1. _____cardium: thick, middle layer of the heart

2. _____cardium: membrane lining the interior wall of the heart

3. _____cardium: thin, outer layer of heart

4. _____cardium: three layer sac that surrounds and protects the heart

5. _____ valves: crescent-shaped cusps through which the ventricles empty

6. _____ valve: located between the right atrium and right ventricle; has three tissue flaps

7. _____ valves: located between the atria and the ventricles

8. _____ valve: located between the left atrium and left ventricle; has two tissue flaps

Part 4 What's in a Name?

Answer the questions in the spaces provided.

1. The reason the coronary arteries received their name: _____

2. The semilunar valves were so named because:_____

3. The name for the sounds created when ventricular filling creates audible vibrations at time of diastole that would be normally silent.

_____

Part 5

Change one word to make the sentence true.

1. Heart valves allow multidirectional flow through the heart.

2. A cardiac output of 4 to 6 LPM is abnormal.

3. The principle arteries that supply heart muscle are the left and retrograde arteries.

4. The endocardium divides the heart into left and right halves.

5. The heart lies between the lungs in the pericardium.

6. The AV node is the normal pacemaker of the heart.

7. Diastole is the period when the atria and ventricles contract.

8. Blood flow through the veins is called microcirculation.

9. The apical pulse is counted at the base of the heart.

10. Chordae tendineae are strands anchored to capillary muscle.

Part 6

Use the information you learned from reading this chapter to provide brief but specific answers to the following instructions.

1. Describe two changes in the conduction system of the heart as a result of aging.

_____

2. Name the atrioventricular (AV) valves and describe their anatomic location.

_____

3. Define Starling's Law.

_____

4. Describe the relationship between the autonomic nerves in the medulla of the brain and the heart.

_____

_____

Part 7 Clinical Thinking

You have just recorded Mrs. Ramos' blood pressure when she nervously asks "Is it all right? The doctor says I have high blood pressure, what does that mean?" In simple words you explain that:

_____
_____
_____
_____
_____
_____

Part 8

Label the structures of the heart on the diagram below.

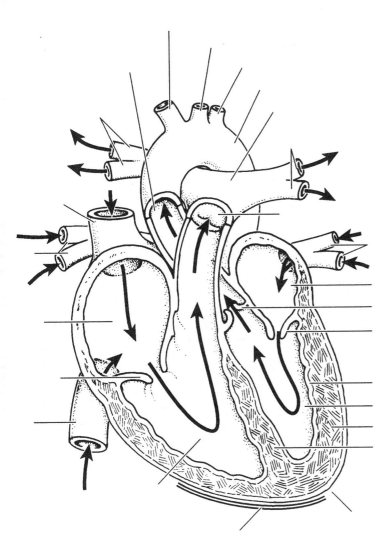

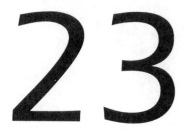

The Hematologic and Lymphatic Systems

Common Acronyms or Terms

B cell

CO_2

Hgb, Hb

Ig

O_2

RBC

Rh

T cell

WBC

CHAPTER OVERVIEW

Chapter 23 outlines the structures of the hematologic and lymphatic systems and describes how they work together to maintain homeostasis in the human body.

✪ Be sure to review the Learning Objectives from the text.

✔ Be sure to FIRST perform Improving Concentration exercises described in the Introduction before proceeding with the next exercise.

PART 1 MATCHING

Indicate which subheading in column I belongs with which major heading in column II.

Column I

1. _____ Lymphatic Circulation
2. _____ Blood
3. _____ Lymph
4. _____ Blood Circulation

Column II

a. Structure and Function

b. System Physiology

c. Effects of Aging on the System

Part 2 Matching

Match the term in column I to the definition in column II.

Column I

1. _____ Thrombocytes
2. _____ Erythrocytes
3. _____ Albumin
4. _____ Hemoglobin
5. _____ Phagocytosis
6. _____ Plasma
7. _____ Lymph nodes
8. _____ Leukocytes
9. _____ Spleen
10. _____ Monocytes
11. _____ Prothrombin
12. _____ Agglutination
13. _____ Globulin
14. _____ Coagulation
15. _____ Tonsils

Column II

a. Agranular leukocytes that are changed to macrophages

b. Largest group of plasma proteins; about 60% to 80%

c. They defend the body against disease, toxins and irritants.

d. Plasma protein made in the liver; carries fat molecules

e. Organ containing lymphoid tissue designed to filter blood

f. Most numerous of the blood cells; disks without a nucleus

g. Blood clotting

h. Clumping of cells; cross-matching checks for this

i. Contained in each RBC, composed of pigment and protein

j. Ring of lymphatic tissue around the pharynx

k. Smallest of the blood's formed elements; platelets

l. Fluid portion of circulating blood

m. Engulfing and destroying invaders; action of some WBCs

n. Plasma protein essential for clotting

o. Small bundles of special lymphoid situated in clusters along lymphatic vessels

Part 3 Multiple Choice

Circle the letter corresponding to the correct answer.

1. The PRIMARY objective of the connective tissue known as blood is to:
   a. Produce and bring red blood cells to maturity
   b. Participate in antibody production to fight foreign invaders
   c. Filter waste products
   d. Maintain a constant environment for the rest of the body tissues
2. The lymphatic organs are all BUT the:
   a. Spleen
   b. Liver
   c. Thymus
   d. Tonsils
3. The pulmonary veins are the only veins that:
   a. Carry nonoxygenated blood
   b. Carry oxygenated blood
   c. Are not unidirectional
   d. Carry blood to the lungs

4. When tissue is injured, platelets break down and cause the release of a chemical called:
   a. Fibrinogen
   b. D factor
   c. Thromboplastin
   d. Prothrombin
5. The most numerous of the white blood cells are the:
   a. Neutrophils
   b. Lymphocytes
   c. Eosinophils
   d. Monocytes

Part 4 True or False

Answer the statements true (T) or false (F).

1. ____ Hematopoiesis originates in the red bone marrow.
2. ____ All white blood cells fight infection.
3. ____ Lymph is a thin, waterless, odorless fluid.
4. ____ Plasma is 70% water.
5. ____ Lymph drains into the lymphatic vessels and then back to veins.
6. ____ Compatible blood can lead to fatal transfusion reactions.
7. ____ The tonsils are an organ of the lymphatic system.
8. ____ Peyer's patches are located in the large intestine.
9. ____ A stationary clot is called a thrombus.
10. ____ The hepatic vein leads to the superior vena cava.
11. ____ The spleen can be removed without ill effects.
12. ____ Blood is considered a connective tissue.
13. ____ Lymph only carries fluid away from tissues.
14. ____ The hepatic portal circulation is unique because it begins and ends with arterioles.
15. ____ Globulin is one of the plasma proteins.

Part 5 The Numbers Game

Choose from the numbers below to make each statement correct.

0	55
80	120
45	1
10	6
4	3
25	

1. Plasma is ____% of the blood volume.

2. The liver and spleen destroy red blood cells in about ____ days.

3. About ____ trillion red blood cells are found in the body.

4. About ____% of the population belongs to blood group AB.

5. Eosinophils can survive up to ____ days.

6. About ____% of Asians and Native Americans are Rh negative.

7. Formed elements comprise ____% of the blood volume.

8. ____% of the population is of the blood group B.

9. The spleen is about ____ inches long.

10. Albumin accounts for up to ____% of the plasma proteins.

Part 6 Discussion

1. State the role of the lymph system in the diagnosis of cancer. _____
_____
_____
_____

2. Explain the term metastasized in relation to the lymph system. _____
_____
_____
_____

24

The Immunologic System

Common Acronyms or Terms

Ab	TF
Ig, IgG, IgM, IgA, IgE, IgD	THF

CHAPTER OVERVIEW

Chapter 24 details the complex defense system the human body uses to protect itself against foreign invasion.

✪ Be sure to review the Learning Objectives from the text.

✔ Be sure to FIRST perform Improving Concentration exercises described in the Introduction before proceeding with the next exercise.

PART 1

Indicate the order in which you would find the following major heading or subheading.

_____ Effects of Aging on the System

_____ Lymphoid Organs

_____ System Physiology

_____ The Mononuclear Phagocyte System

_____ Types of Specific Immunity

Part 2 Multiple Choice

Circle the letter corresponding to the correct answer.

1. A complement is a group of proteins normally present, but inactive in the:
   a. Bone marrow
   b. Lymph
   c. Blood
   d. Thymus

2. IgE is one of the immunoglobulins that:
   a. Protects the fetus before birth
   b. Is responsible for allergic reactions
   c. Protects mucosal surfaces
   d. Stimulates complement activity

3. The thymus is located in the:
   a. Mediastinum
   b. Medulla
   c. Mid pons
   d. Marrow

4. Macrophages destroy:
   a. B cells
   b. Antigens
   c. Antibodies
   d. T cells

5. Monocytes are agranular and so are:
   a. Neutrophils
   b. Basophils
   c. Lymphocytes
   d. Eosinophils

Part 3

Change one word to make the sentence true.

1. T cells mature in the bone marrow.

2. Antibodies destroy antigens.

3. Cell-mediated immunity refers to the destruction of antigens by B cells.

4. Radial immunity refers to destruction of antigens by antibodies.

5. T lymphocytes are responsible for tissue acceptance after organ transplantation.

6. Bone marrow and the thymus are considered secondary lymphoid organs.

7. Dust cells are located in the liver.

8. Interleukins retard T-cell growth.

9. Antibodies are substances the immune system recognizes as foreign.

10. The thymus gland begins to enlarge at puberty.

Part 4

Complete the sentence by filling in the blank.

1. _____ is a protein made by several types of cells that inhibits virus production and infection.

2. _____ are also called antibodies and gamma globulins.

3. Bone marrow is responsible for the production and maturation of _____ lymphocytes.

4. Nonspecific immunity is one of the body's _____ systems.

5. Autoimmune diseases can occur if the immune system is _____.

Part 5 Clinical Thinking

Mrs. Jackson has just given birth to her first child. She asks you the advantages of breast milk over formula. Strictly from an immunologic viewpoint you explain the role of breast milk in relation to an infant's immune system. What would you tell her?

_____

_____

_____

_____

_____

_____

_____

25

The Respiratory System

Common Acronyms or Terms

CO	O_2
CO_2	RV
ERV	TLC
H_2CO_3	TV
IRV	VC

CHAPTER OVERVIEW

Chapter 25 details the anatomy and physiology of normal respiration and the effects of aging on the respiratory system.

✪ Be sure to review the Learning Objectives from the text.

✔ Be sure to FIRST perform Improving Concentration exercises described in the Introduction before proceeding with the next exercise.

Part 1

Complete the following statements by filling in the blanks.

1. The first subheadings under each major heading are: _____, _____, _____, and _____.

2. The major heading that has no subheadings is _____.

Part 2 Multiple Choice

Circle the letter corresponding to the correct answer and state the heading under which the answer is located.

1. Choose the statement that is *not* a natural effect of aging.
   a. Lungs become less elastic.
   b. Chest walls become stiffer.
   c. Alveoli may collapse due to insufficient surfactant.
   d. Mucous secretion in the lining of the respiratory tract decreases.

2. The exchange of gas at the cellular level is called:
   a. Internal respiration
   b. External respiration
   c. Inspiration
   d. Ventilation

3. The primary function of the respiratory system is:
   a. Gas exchange
   b. Mucous production
   c. Regulation of body pH
   d. Production of sound from vocal cords

4. The sinuses drain directly into the:
   a. Throat
   b. Nasal cavities
   c. Trachea
   d. Bronchi

5. Normal respiration is called:
   a. Dyspnea
   b. Apnea
   c. Eupnea
   d. Tachypnea

Part 3

Using words from the key terms complete the following sentences.

1. The process by which oxygen is exchanged for carbon dioxide within the alveoli of the lungs is called _____ _____.

2. The _____ are located between the ribs; they contract to lift and spread the ribs during inhalation.

3. _____ _____ is the amount of air inspired or expired during normal respiration.

4. The exchange of oxygen for carbon dioxide within the cells (cell breathing) is also known as _____ or _____.

5. _____ _____ is the maximum amount of air that can be exhaled following a maximum inhalation.

Part 4 True or False

Answer these statements true (T) or false (F) and correct the false.

1. _____ The trachea and pharynx are both located in the esophagus.

2. _____ The pleura has three layers.

3. _____ The pharynx is divided into three parts.

4. _____ Internal respiration is exchange of gas at the lung level.

5. _____ Sneezing and coughing are protective reflexes of the respiratory system.

Part 5

Choose from the word list below to supply the correct term for the given definition.

1. Dome-shaped muscle that separates the thorax and the abdomen _____

2. Box-like structure made of cartilage _____

3. The bronchioles branch first into these, which look like stems. _____

4. Point at which the arteries, veins, bronchi, and nerves enter the lungs _____

5. Tonsils are located in this area, commonly called the throat. _____

6. The space between the two layers of the pleura where a vacuum normally exists _____

7. The lowest portion of the pharynx _____

8. The top of each of the cone-shaped lungs _____

9. Respiratory center that automatically controls the rate and depth of respiration _____

10. Protective flap that covers the trachea during swallowing _____

Epiglottis

Medulla

Pleural cavity

Diaphragm

Larynx

Apex

Laryngopharynx

Alveolar ducts

Oropharynx

Hilum

26

The Digestive System

Common Acronyms or Terms

ATP

CHO

CHL

GI

CHAPTER OVERVIEW

Chapter 26 details the anatomy and physiology of the digestive system and the effects of aging.

✪ Be sure to review the Learning Objectives from the text.

✔ Be sure to FIRST perform Improving Concentration exercises described in the Introduction before proceeding with the next exercise.

PART 1

Using information found in the major headings and key terms change one word to make the sentence true.

1. The digestive tract is open to the outside on both ends and is sterile.

2. The first portion of the small intestine is the C-shaped jejunum.

3. The gallbladder is the body's largest glandular organ.

4. Most nutrient absorption occurs in the large intestine.

5. The large intestine produces vitamin C and B complex vitamins.

Part 2

Match the term in column I to the definition in column II.

Column I

1. _____ Entero

2. _____ Digestion

3. _____ Bile

4. _____ Anabolism

5. _____ Mastication

6. _____ Deglutition

7. _____ Villi

8. _____ Defecation

9. _____ Peritoneum

10. _____ Catabolism

Column II

a. Large sheet of serous membrane: covers abdominal organs

b. Breaking food into small particles: chewing

c. Destructive metabolism

d. Finger-like projections of the intestine

e. Process of eliminating intestinal wastes

f. Constructive metabolism

g. Prefix referring to the intestines

h. Conversion of food to usable material for energy

i. Beginning of the swallowing process

j. Liquid made by the liver and stored in the gallbladder

Part 3

Name the labeled components of the digestive system.

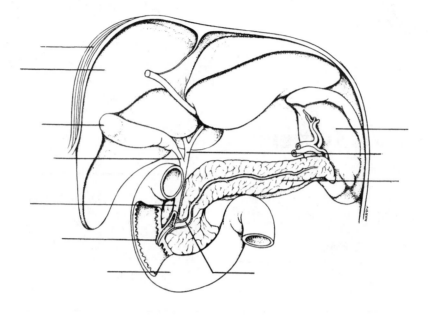

Part 4 Multiple Choice

Circle the letter corresponding to the correct answer.

1. The conversion of food into substances that can be easily absorbed is:
   a. Mechanical digestion
   b. Chemical digestion
   c. Deglutition
   d. Mastication

2. The first portion of the large intestine is the:
   a. Duodenum
   b. Jejunum
   c. Ileum
   d. Cecum

3. The digestive process begins in the:
   a. Large intestine
   b. Small intestine
   c. Stomach
   d. Mouth

4. The substance in dead-end lymph capillaries within each villus is:
   a. Amylase
   b. Trypsin
   c. Chyle
   d. Lipase

5. Basal metabolism refers to:
   a. The amount of calories the body uses at rest
   b. The breakdown of larger molecules into smaller ones
   c. The breakdown of the chemical bonds in food
   d. The transfer of food into the circulation for transport

Part 5 Clinical Thinking

Mrs. Ferguson has a history of gallbladder disease. After you deliver her breakfast, she lifts the cover and sighs, "I sure would like a good old-fashioned breakfast of bacon and eggs and homefries. Nurse, why can't I get some real food around here?"

From a physiology viewpoint, explain the role of the gallbladder in normal fat absorption and emulsification.

_____

_____

_____

_____

_____

_____

27

The Urinary System

Common Acronyms or Terms

ADH

ANP

BUN

cm

CHAPTER OVERVIEW

Chapter 27 reviews the normal anatomy and physiology of the urinary system and the effects of aging.

✪ Be sure to review the Learning Objectives from the text.

✍ Be sure to FIRST perform Improving Concentration exercises described in the Introduction before proceeding with the next exercise.

Part 1

Complete the following statements related to the major headings and key points.

1. The second heading under "Structure and Function" is: _____.

2. The two headings under "System Physiology" discuss _____ _____ and _____.

3. The urinary system eliminates _____, controls water _____, regulates _____ levels, maintains _____ balance, activates vitamin _____, and secretes _____ and _____.

Part 2 True or False

Answer these statements true (T) or (F) false. Correct the false.

1. _____ Nephrons are the functional unit of the kidney responsible for expelling urine.

2. _____ Renal blood is highly oxygenated because it comes directly from the aorta.

3. _____ The urinary bladder is a reservoir that forms urine.

4. _____ The number and size of nephrons normally decrease after age 40.

5. _____ Urine is normally about 75% water.

6. _____ Anatomically, the kidneys normally lie anterior to the peritoneum.

7. _____ The kidneys secrete a hormone called erythropoietin.

8. _____ The loops of Henle are located in the renal cortex.

9. _____ Approximately 50% of the circulating blood volume circulates through the kidneys daily.

10. _____ The glomeruli complete the process of the secretion of urine.

Part 3

Supply the correct term for the following definitions.

1. _____
   Release of urine from the body, also called voiding

2. _____
   Medical term that means "behind the peritoneum"

3. _____
   Functional unit of the kidney

4. _____
   Hormone secreted by the kidney important in blood pressure regulation

5. _____
   Accumulation of water in the tissues

6. _____
   Process in which a cell ingests substances

7. _____
   Waking up to void at night

8. _____
   Tubes attached to the kidneys at the renal pelvis that carry urine to the bladder

9. _____
   Renal hormone that stimulates red bone marrow during hypoxia

10. _____
    Urine is composed of 95% of this substance.

Part 4 Critical Thinking

Before you empty Mr. Rosen's urinal you note several things prior to discarding it. State what you would take note of and why.

Part 5 The Numbers Game

Using the list of numbers below, complete the following statements.

1. The average length of the urethra in men is _____ inches.

2. A bladder can hold more than _____ liter of fluid.

3. The kidneys are about _____ inches long.

4. Urine is about _____% solutes.

5. The average female urethra is less than _____ inches long.

1

2

4

5

8

28

The Male Reproductive System

Common Acronyms or Terms

FSH

ICSH

CHAPTER OVERVIEW

Chapter 28 discusses the normal anatomy and physiology and the effects of aging on the male reproductive system.

✪ Be sure to review the Learning Objectives from the text.

✍ Be sure to FIRST perform Improving Concentration exercises described in the Introduction before proceeding with the next exercise.

Part 1 Multiple Choice

Using information from the key points, circle the letter corresponding to the correct answer.

1. Male hormones are called:
   a. Spermatozoa
   b. Gonads
   c. Androgens
   d. Estrogens

2. The sac that supports and protects the testes is the:
   a. Ductus deferens
   b. Scrotum
   c. Epididymis
   d. Prostate

3. The main male androgen is:
   a. Progesterone
   b. Testosterone
   c. Spermatozoa
   d. Estrogen

4. Sperm cells are stored in the:
   a. Ductus deferens
   b. Scrotum
   c. Epididymis
   d. Prostate

5. This organ serves as the common passageway for both the urinary and reproductive systems.
   a. Gonads
   b. Testes
   c. Genitals
   d. Penis

6. The major heading that contains subheadings titled "Testes and Accessory Glands" is:
   a. Hormonal Influences
   b. Structure and Function
   c. System Physiology
   d. Effects on Aging on the System

Part 2

Using words from the list of key terms complete the sentences.

1. The male gonads, stimulated by _____, form sperm.

2. The _____ is a doughnut-shaped muscular organ that lies just below the bladder.

3. During _____ the penis becomes firm to penetrate the vagina.

4. The _____ produce sperm cells and secrete sex hormones.

5. Surgical removal of the prepuce is called _____.

Part 3 True or False

Answer these statements true (T) or false (F). Correct the false.

1. _____ Men stop producing sperm at a phase called andropause.

2. _____ Cowper's glands are about the size of a pea and are located superior to the prostate.

3. _____ The head of a sperm cell contains 23 chromosomes.

4. _____ Prepuce is another name for foreskin.

5. _____ Nocturnal emissions in pubescent boys are normal.

Part 4 Clinical Thinking

You are assigned to care for a 36-year-old client, immediately after outpatient surgery for bilateral inguinal hernia repair. Although you do not know the patient's name or gender you are aware that men are more likely to experience this type of hernia because:

_____

_____

_____

_____

_____

_____

29

The Female Reproductive System

Common Acronyms or Terms

ERT

FSH

LH

CHAPTER OVERVIEW

Chapter 29 reviews the normal anatomy and physiology of the female reproductive system and also discusses the effects of aging.

✪ Be sure to review the Learning Objectives from the text.

✔ Be sure to FIRST perform Improving Concentration exercises described in the Introduction before proceeding with the next exercise.

Part 1

Determine under what heading you would find more information about the following topics:

Oviducts _____

Physical changes associated with growing older

_____

Part 2

Choosing words from the key terms complete the following sentences.

1. The external structure of the female genitalia that is a fatty pad over the symphysis pubis is

   _____.

2. If the ovum is not fertilized, secretion of _____ decreases and the corpus luteum begins to decline.

3. These vestibular glands that lubricate the vagina are also called _____.

4. Each _____ develops in different stages throughout a woman's life.

5. Luteinizing and follicle-stimulating hormone stimulated by the hypothalamus are considered

   _____.

Part 3 The Numbers Game

Choose a number from the list below to correctly complete the sentence.

1. During pregnancy the uterus increases its size about ____ times.

2. Menses occurs about every ____ days.

3. The nonpregnant uterus is about ____ inches wide.

4. Ovulation occurs around day ____ (the middle) of the menstrual cycle.

5. The uterus has ____ layers.

2	6
3	28
14	

Part 4

Change one word to make the statement true.

1. The egg cell is called a zygote.
2. Menarche is the time when the menstrual periods cease.
3. Female hormones are called androgens.
4. The mammary glands function to produce and to release milk before childbirth.
5. Fertilization of the ovum occurs in the uterus.
6. The internal genitalia are collectively called the vulva.
7. The female perineum is the space between the vaginal orifice and the urethra.
8. The mucous layer of the uterus is called the myometrium.
9. The ruptured graafian follicle becomes the corpus luteum during the follicular phase.
10. The oviducts enter the uterus at its upper end called the cervix.

Part 5 Matched Pairs

Each term in column I is related to another term in column II. Draw a line from one related term to the other.

Column I

Ovary

Painful intercourse

Zygote

Oviduct

Mature oocyte

Uterus

Clitoris

Column II

Fallopian tube

Womb

Penis

Gonad

Ovum

Dyspareunia

Fertilized ovum

30

Basic Nutrition

Common Acronyms or Terms

ADA	Kcal
BMI	LDL
C	NE
CHO	PCM
DRI	PKU
EAR	RDA
ESADDI	RE
Fe	REE
GI	TE
HDL	UL
HFCS	USDA
IF	

CHAPTER OVERVIEW

Chapter 30 addresses nutrition and the necessary nutrients for health and wellness across the life span. An overview of common nutritional problems and their impact on wellness is provided.

✪ Be sure to review the Learning Objectives from the text.

✍ Be sure to FIRST perform Improving Concentration exercises described in the Introduction before proceeding with the next exercise.

Part 1

Indicate if the following subheadings are located under the major heading: **Nutrients—N, A Healthy Diet—HD, or Nutrition Across the Life Span—NAL.**

1. _____ Enzymes and Digestion

2. _____ Nutritional Problems

3. _____ Early and Middle Adulthood

4. _____ Pregnancy

5. _____ Recommended Dietary Allowances

Part 2

Complete the word for the definition provided.

1. R_____
   D_____
   A_____
   Daily amount of nutrients considered adequate in meeting the nutritional needs of practically all Americans

2. E_____
   C_____
   An imprecise term applied to foods that supply calories with few or no nutrients; candy, soft drinks

3. E_____
   N_____
   Substances needed for growth that must be obtained through food; the body cannot make these in sufficient quantity.

4. N_____
   D_____
   Foods that provide significant amounts of key nutrients per volume consumed

5. B_____
   M_____
   I_____
   Method of measuring obesity; weight divided by height

6. R_____
   E_____
   E_____
   The total calories needed to keep body processes going

7. E_____
Biologic catalysts made of proteins

8. K_____
The unit of measurement that specifies the heat energy in a particular amount of food; heat required to raise the temperature of 1 kg of water 1°C

9. E_____ requirements
Total calories needed to keep body processes going and to carry on physical activities

10. M_____
Too much or too little of one or more nutrients; bad nutrition

Part 3

Match the nutrient in column I with the nutrient source in column II and the major function of the nutrient in column III.

Column I

1. _____ Carbohydrate

2. _____ Fat

3. _____ Protein

Column II

a. Butter, cream, and avocado

b. Meat, milk, and cheese

c. Potato, lima beans, and corn

Column III

d. Carries vitamins A, D, E, and K

e. Builds and repairs all tissues, including blood

f. Major source of energy (glucose)

Part 4 Short Answer Exercises

Complete the following questions by filling in the blanks.

1. Our understanding of the role of nutrition has shifted from simply _____ dietary deficiencies to _____ the _____ of chronic illness and in the future perhaps _____ health.

2. The six classes of nutrients include carbohydrates, fats, protein, _____, _____, and _____.

3. _____ is so necessary to life nature has provided human beings with an inborn warning device; _____ is our strongest appetite.

4. _____ are vital for building bones and teeth, maintaining muscle tone, regulating body processes, and maintaining acid–base balance.

5. _____ are comprised of carbon, oxygen, hydrogen, and sometimes nitrogen or other elements.

6. A person who is more than 10% over desirable weight for body frame is considered _____; a person 20% above desired weight is considered to be _____.

Part 5

Indicate if the following actions would be appropriate (A) or inappropriate (I) to promote good nutrition.

1. _____ Encourage the pregnant woman to consume 50% more calories during the second and third trimesters than before her pregnancy.

2. _____ Instruct new mothers to feed infants every 3 hours to promote routine and improve digestion.

3. _____ Inform women who wish to become pregnant that intake of folic acid, protein, iron, calcium, and vitamin D are especially important.

4. _____ Teach parents of toddlers that children should be allowed to eat to satisfy hunger because appetite fluctuates widely with growth patterns.

5. _____ Adolescents should be provided specific foods at meals and for snacks to prevent snacking and meals with empty calories such as junk foods.

6. _____ Inform early and middle adulthood clients that caloric requirements may decrease because the individual is no longer growing.

7. ____ Assess individuals in older adulthood for economic difficulties or poor dental status that may result in poor nutritional intake.

8. ____ Encourage all individuals to eat more protein and fewer carbohydrates to decrease calorie intake.

Part 6

Answer these statements true (T) or false (F). Correct the false.

1. ____ Iron is important to form bone and regulate nerves.

2. ____ Calcium promotes blood clotting and provides muscle function.

3. ____ Phosphorous acts in acid–base balance and energy metabolism.

4. ____ Vitamin D is water soluble; it is also known as ascorbic acid.

5. ____ Vitamin A maintains normal vision and helps the eye to adapt to dim light.

Part 7 Multiple Choice

Circle the letter corresponding to the correct answer.

1. Elaine is 30 years old and 5 feet, 6 inches tall with an average body frame. Based on the formula in your text, what would Elaine's ideal body weight be?
   a. 122 pounds
   b. 130 pounds
   c. 136 pounds
   d. 142 pounds

2. Using Table 30-8 in your text, an individual who weighs 190 pounds and is 5 feet, 9 inches tall has a body mass index of:
   a. 28
   b. 30
   c. 31
   d. 37

3. While teaching a 12th grade class about nutrition and healthy eating you would be sure to include that:
   a. Overnutrition is not possible in teen years because energy expenditure is so high.
   b. Teenagers do not get atherosclerosis so they should not worry about saturated fats.
   c. The nutritional problems of most Americans are due to deficiencies of proteins.
   d. Overnutrition contributes to such conditions as hypertension and osteoporosis.

4. Niketa is 2 years old and her mother tells you "I know she needs to eat more." You should suggest to the mother:
   a. Fill Niketa's plate each meal then encourage seconds.
   b. Insist that Niketa should "clean her plate" each meal.
   c. Not worry as long as Niketa has reasonable intake from each major food group.
   d. Provide Niketa with privacy during meals, particularly when she is eating hot dogs or grapes.

Part 8

Label the following illustration by placing the correct letter by the titles provided.

1. Fruits   _____
2. Vegetables   _____
3. Meat   _____
4. Milk   _____
5. Grain   _____
6. Other (fats, sweets) _____

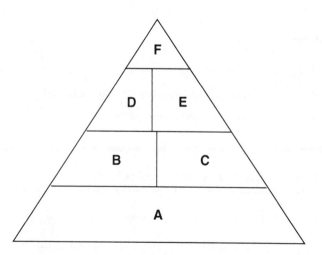

31

Transcultural and Social Aspects of Nutrition

CHAPTER OVERVIEW

Chapter 31 discusses cultural and other social influences on nutrition. Dietary practices common to various cultural groups are addressed. Concerns related to social factors that affect food choices are also discussed.

✪ Be sure to review the Learning Objectives from the text.

✔ Be sure to FIRST perform Improving Concentration exercises described in the Introduction before proceeding with the next exercise.

Part 1

Complete the following titles of some major headings in the chapter.

1. The V_____ C_____

2. R_____
   B_____

3. R_____
   P_____

4. E_____
   H_____

Part 2

Complete the following statements by filling in the blanks.

1. To provide optimum care, understand the _____ aspects of food and eating and work within a person's cultural context.

2. _____ and _____ factors may play an important part in food acceptance.

3. Pure vegans may need vitamin ____ and vitamin ____ supplements.

Part 3

Unscramble the letters to reveal the word defined below the line.

1. Skehor _____
   Separate dishes are used to prepare and serve meat and dairy foods; pork, shellfish, and rabbit are not allowed.

2. Fout _____
   Soybean curd

3. Luso odfo _____
   Both cooking style and particular foods, such as black-eyed peas and collard greens

4. Clota-voo _____ vegetarian
   Individual eats plant foods, dairy products and eggs

Part 4

Indicate if the following action would be appropriate (A) or inappropriate (I) to help clients with transcultural or social food pattern influences meet nutritional needs.

1. _____ Encouraging intake of dairy products by persons who have lactose intolerance to meet their calcium needs

2. _____ Instructing clients to boil vegetables for long periods of time to improve texture and vitamin content

3. _____ Assisting African American clients in planning meals to reduce sodium, fat, and sugar to prevent chronic illnesses

4. _____ Discussing the need for lacto-ovo vegetarians to eat the same plant proteins from day to day to maintain protein levels

5. _____ Placing clients in rooms or areas with other clients at meal time to encourage intake

6. _____ Serving ham and shellfish to a client who is an Orthodox Jew

7. _____ Serving tea or coffee with the meal for a client who is Islamic or Muslim

8. _____ Stressing adequate nutrient intake over a low-fat or low-calorie diet when nutritional needs are increased because of illness or injury

9. _____ Requesting a diet with no meat for the meals on Friday for a client who is Roman Catholic

10. _____ Initiating a referral to social services for a client who does not have money for food

Part 5

Match the dietary practices and concerns in column I with the appropriate ethnic group in column II.

Column I

1. _____ Limited use of meats; malt beer may be given to children

2. _____ Believes in the Yin (cold)–Yang (hot) concept of balancing intake

3. _____ Milk is rarely used after childhood.

4. _____ Calcium and protein intake may be inadequate.

5. _____ Food has great religious and social significance; milk is seldom used.

Column II

a. Asian Americans—Chinese

b. Native Americans

c. Puerto Rican

d. South Asian

e. Middle Eastern

32

Diet Therapy and Special Diets

Common Acronyms or Terms

FF

G tube

I & O

IV

J tube

Na

Ng

NPO

PEG

STAT

TPN

CHAPTER OVERVIEW

Chapter 32 discusses nutritional support for clients with various conditions. Modified diets and the nurse's role in providing nutritional support for clients are addressed. The use of tube feedings and parenteral nutrition are discussed.

✪ Be sure to review the Learning Objectives from the text.

✔ Be sure to FIRST perform Improving Concentration exercises described in the Introduction before proceeding with the next exercise.

Part 1

In what order would you find the following major headings in the chapter?

1. _____ The Client Who Needs Assistance With Eating

2. _____ Nutritional Support

3. _____ Helping the Client Meet Nutritional Needs

4. _____ House Diets

5. _____ Food and Medication Interactions

6. _____ Modified Diets

Part 2

Answer these statements true (T) or false (F) based on your review of the major headings and key points.

1. _____ Too much plain water can lead to electrolyte imbalance.

2. _____ Diet progression for diet as tolerated begins with soft foods, then liquids to prevent choking.

3. _____ Tube feeding is a commonly used means of providing nourishment.

4. _____ "Encouraging Fluid Intake" is a subheading under the major heading "Helping the Client Meet Nutritional Needs."

Part 3 Key Terms: Knowledge Check

Review the key terms in the chapter. Most of following definitions or statements are incorrect. Correct the word(s), when needed, to make all definitions/statements accurate.

1. _____ diets are composed of food with extra fiber to clear the residue from the intestines.

2. _____ diets are often used to treat individuals with _____ blood lipids.

3. Fried foods _____ acceptable in bland diets because the goal of the diet is to decrease gastric acid production.

4. Soft diets are nutritionally adequate and are _____ in fiber, connective tissue, and fat.

5. The _____ is based on the Diabetic Exchange Lists for Meal Planning.

6. _____ is a specifically formulated solution, nutritionally complete, that is used when the gastrointestinal tract is functioning.

Part 4

Fill in term or terms that best match(es) the definition.

1. _____
   Medical term for a swallowing disorder

2. _____
   Elevated blood lipids

3. _____
   Loss of appetite

4. _____
   Excess accumulation of water and salts in tissues

5. _____
   Contains lesser concentrations of the same ingredients found in central vein TPN

Part 5

Match the list of diet types in column I with the classification of diet modifications in column II.

Column I

1. _____ Liquid, soft, high-fiber, low-residue, and bland diets

2. _____ High calorie, low calorie

3. _____ High- and low-fat; protein, sodium, calcium, or potassium controlled

4. _____ Six small feedings per day

5. _____ "No eggs or no milk on trays"

Column II

a. Nutrients

b. Specific allergens

c. Consistency and texture

d. Energy value

e. Amount

Part 6 Skill Drill

Order the following steps in administering a tube feeding.

1. _____ Position the client with the head of the bed elevated.

2. _____ Hang the feeding bag set up 12 to 18 inches.

3. _____ Explain the procedure to the client.

4. _____ Add 30 to 60 mL water to the feeding bag as feeding is complete.

5. _____ Determine placement of feeding tube; aspirate stomach secretions or inject air and listen for gurgling.

6. _____ Prepare formula.

33

Introduction to the Nursing Process

CHAPTER OVERVIEW

Chapter 33 discusses the nursing process and the concepts of problem-solving and critical thinking. The nurse's role in each step of the nursing process is addressed.

✪ Be sure to review the Learning Objectives from the text.

✔ Be sure to FIRST perform Improving Concentration exercises described in the Introduction before proceeding with the next exercise.

Part 1

In what order would you find the following major headings or subheadings in the chapter?

1. _____ Characteristics of the Nursing Process

2. _____ Problem-Solving

3. _____ Steps in the Nursing Process

4. _____ Critical Thinking

5. _____ Nursing Process

Part 2

Answer these statements true (T) or false (F) based on your review of the major headings and key points.

1. _____ Scientists have used scientific problem-solving for many years to systematize their research.

2. _____ The nursing process cannot be used to provide individualized care that is accountable.

3. _____ The client and the family should be involved in the nursing care plan after it is developed and implementation is begun.

4. _____ "The Nursing Process and Quality Care" is a major heading in this chapter.

Part 3 Key Terms: Knowledge Check

Review the key terms in the chapter. Complete the statements to make all definitions/statements accurate.

1. _____ is experimental problem-solving that tests ideas to decide which methods work and which do not.

2. _____ is use of a complicated mix of inquiry, knowledge, intuition, logic, experience, and common sense to solve a problem.

3. As a nurse, you combine critical thinking with a scientific problem-solving method to identify and address client problems; this framework for thinking and acting is called the

_____ _____.

4. Nursing care that is focused on the individual client's needs and not just on performing skills or tasks is considered _____

_____.

5. Guidelines developed when caring for each client, to ensure consistency among all nursing staff, are called _____ _____

_____.

Part 4

Fill in the specific step of the nursing process in which the nurse would perform the identified acts.

1. _____
   Write a nursing care plan (NCP)

2. _____
   Plan for future nursing care; revise plan as needed

3. _____
   Identify assessment priorities; collect data

4. _____
   Put NCP into action; continue collecting data

5. _____
   Recognize significant data; recognize patterns or clusters

Part 5

Match the steps of scientific problem-solving in column I with the related steps in the nursing process in column II.

Column I

1. _____ Formulate tentative solutions; choose preferred solutions

2. _____ Evaluate the results; formulate another tentative solution

3. _____ Gather information relative to the problem

4. _____ Identify the problem

5. _____ Test solutions

Column II

a. Nursing assessment

b. Nursing diagnosis

c. Nursing planning

d. Nursing implementation

e. Nursing evaluation

Part 6 Short Answer

Explain briefly how critical thinking relates to problem-solving.

_____

_____

_____

_____

_____

_____

34

Nursing Assessment

Common Acronyms or Terms

ADLs   CC

CHAPTER OVERVIEW

Chapter 34 explores first step of the nursing process, assessment. Types and methods of data collection are discussed, and the process of data analysis is addressed.

✪ Be sure to review the Learning Objectives from the text.

✔ Be sure to FIRST perform Improving Concentration exercises described in the Introduction before proceeding with the next exercise.

Part 1

Match the headings in column I with the major headings in this chapter under which they may be found in column II.

Column I

1. _____ Identifying Strengths and Analyzing Problems
2. _____ Types of Data Collection
3. _____ Validating Observations
4. _____ Recognizing Patterns or Clusters
5. _____ Types of Data Collection

Column II

a. Nursing Assessment
b. Data Analysis

Part 2

Fill in the term or terms that best match(es) the definition.

1. _____
   _____
   All the measurable and observable pieces of information about a client, such as vital signs

2. _____
   _____
   A way of soliciting information from the client, also called a nursing history

3. _____
   Assessment tool that relies on the use of the five senses to discover objective information about the client

4. _____
   _____
   Consist of the client's opinions or feelings about what is happening

5. _____
   _____
   Assist you in drawing conclusions regarding the client's health problems; critical thinking skills used

Part 3

Match the data collection method described in column I with the most accurate title listed in column II.

Column I

1. _____ Touching or palpating the skin to determine temperature
2. _____ Obtaining biographical data from the client or a family member
3. _____ Examining the client's body
4. _____ Noting if the client has a body odor
5. _____ Inquiring about the client's activities of daily living

Column II

a. Physical examination
b. Observation
c. Interview

Part 4 Short Answer Exercises

Complete the following short answer questions.

1. Briefly list and describe the steps in data analysis.

   _____

   _____

2. Nursing assessment is the systematic and continuous _____ and _____ of information about the client.

3. The best sources of information about the client are the _____ and _____.

Part 5 Multiple Choice

Circle the letter corresponding to the correct answer.

1. Jene McInerny, age 29, is admitted for complaints of numbness in her legs alternating with weakness. Which of the following represents a question the nurse might ask in the client interview that is most closely related to the client's complaint?
   a. "Do you have any speech problems?"
   b. "Are you sexually active and do you have any sexual concerns?"
   c. "Do you need to see someone from social services?"
   d. "Do you have any problems walking by yourself, or do you need assistance?"

2. Which of the following would be subjective data?
   a. The client's blood pressure is 130/58.
   b. Client states pain is at an intensity of 8 out of 10.
   c. Client has blue coloring at the fingertips and under her fingernails.
   d. The client's respirations are shallow and nonlabored.

35

Diagnosing and Planning

Common Acronyms or Terms

AEB

NANDA

NCP

POC

PRN

R/T

CHAPTER OVERVIEW

Chapter 35 explores the diagnosing and planning steps in the nursing process. Nursing diagnoses are addressed including a discussion of the differences between nursing and medical diagnoses. The process of writing nursing diagnoses and planning care related to those diagnoses is discussed.

✪ Be sure to review the Learning Objectives from the text.

✔ Be sure to FIRST perform Improving Concentration exercises described in the Introduction before proceeding with the next exercise.

Part 1

Match the headings in column I with the major headings in this chapter under which they may be found in column II.

Column I

1. _____ Selecting Nursing Interventions

2. _____ Setting Priorities

3. _____ Writing a Diagnostic Statement

4. _____ NANDA-Approved Nursing Diagnoses

5. _____ Writing a Nursing Care Plan

Column II

a. Nursing Diagnosis

b. Planning Care

Part 2

Unscramble the letters, then fill in the term or terms that best match(es) the definition.

1. Depetcex mucoteo _____

_____

A measurable client behavior that indicates whether the person has achieved the expected benefit of nursing care

2. Damile andissogi _____

Identifies the disease a person has or is believed to have and provides a basis for prognosis and medical treatment decisions

3. Runnisg isangisod _____

Statement about a client's actual or potential health concerns that can be managed through independent nursing interventions

4. Daxerk _____
A flip-file with card slots or a notebook for each client on a unit or nursing care team

5. Blolatrovicae morpleb _____

_____

Means that the nurse will work with the physician or other healthcare providers

Part 3

*Indicate if the following diagnoses are **nursing diagnoses (N) or medical diagnoses (M).***

1. _____ Ineffective Airway Clearance

2. _____ Pneumonia

3. _____ Hyperthermia

4. _____ Pain

5. _____ Diabetes

Part 4 Short Answer Exercises

Complete these short answer questions by filling in the blanks.

1. The three components of a nursing diagnosis are the p_____ (diagnostic label), e_____(cause), and s_____ and s_____.

2. List and describe how the nurse carries out the steps in planning client care. _____
_____

Part 5

Prioritize the following nursing diagnoses as primary (P), secondary (S), or tertiary (T) based on hierarchy of needs.

1. _____ *Risk for Injury* related to unsteady gait

2. _____ *Fluid Volume Deficit*

3. _____ *Altered Self-Esteem*

4. _____ *Anxiety*

5. _____ *Altered Role Performance*

6. _____ *Ineffective Airway Clearance*

36

Implementing and Evaluating Care

CHAPTER OVERVIEW

Chapter 36 discusses the steps in carrying out nursing interventions (implementation) and determining the effectiveness of those interventions (evaluation). Nursing skills are addressed, including communication and data collection skills. Analysis of client responses to care and factors that might contribute to those responses are discussed as steps in the evaluation of nursing care and planning of future nursing care.

✪ Be sure to review the Learning Objectives from the text.

✔ Be sure to FIRST perform Improving Concentration exercises described in the Introduction before proceeding with the next exercise.

Part 1

Match the headings in column I with the major headings in this chapter under which they may be found in column II.

Column I

1. _____ Skills Used in Nursing
2. _____ Planning Future Nursing Care
3. _____ The Chart Audit
4. _____ Continuing Collection of Data
5. _____ Identifying Factors Contributing to Success or Failure
6. _____ Nursing Peer Review

Column II

a. Evaluating Nursing Care
b. Implementing Care
c. Quality Assurance
d. Discharge Planning

Part 2

Fill in term or terms that best match(es) the definition.

1. _____
   Step in the nursing process in which you carry out the plan

2. _____
   Actions that carry out a physician's orders regarding medication or treatments

3. _____
   Responsibility for all actions the nurse performs

4. _____
   Skills used in nursing that involve believing, behaving, and relating

5. _____
   Skills in nursing that involve knowing and understanding essential information

6. _____
   Measuring client outcomes, examining all aspects of healthcare organization, evaluating overall effectiveness through voluntary surveys from outside accreditation agencies, and conducting performance evaluations to rate care provided by the facility itself

7. _____
   Evaluation of outcomes of care from the client's viewpoint

8. _____
   Evaluation of nursing activities and client outcomes as they are demonstrated in the nursing documentation

Part 3

Match the following terms or concepts in column I with the related statements in column II.

Column I

1. _____ Evaluation

2. _____ Independent actions

3. _____ Variance

4. _____ Discharge planning

5. _____ Case manager

6. _____ Interdependent actions

7. _____ Clinical care path

8. _____ Technical skills

Column II

a. Actions that you perform collaboratively with other care providers

b. Actions such as changing a sterile dressing or administering an injection

c. Plans and directs all necessary activities to coordinate the client's care

d. Measurement of effectiveness of assessing, diagnosing, planning, and implementing

e. Planning method in which the optimal sequencing and timing of healthcare interventions are identified

f. Occurs in a clinical care path if a client does not achieve an expected outcome by the designated time

g. Nursing actions that do not require a physician's orders

h. Process by which the client is prepared for continued care outside the healthcare facility

Part 4 Short Answer Exercises

Complete the following short answer questions.

1. The action phrases of implementation include *doing* nursing care; _____ with clients and members of the healthcare team; and _____ information so the next healthcare provider can act.

2. List steps in evaluating the effectiveness of nursing care. _____

_____

Part 5

Circle the letter corresponding to the correct answer.

1. James Gey has had hip replacement surgery. The doctor wrote an order for pain medication as needed. You observe Mr. Gey has a frown and grimace on his face and is holding his hip. You ask if he is hurting and after he states his pain level is a 9 out of 10 you administer pain medication. The above describes a(n) _____ nursing action.
   a. Independent
   b. Dependent
   c. Interdependent
   d. Interpersonal

2. Jean RN has implemented a clinical care path for Mr. Phong, a client admitted with advanced-stage cancer. To determine the effectiveness of the care provided Mr. Phong, which of the following actions would *not* be a step in the evaluation of nursing care?
   a. Ask the client and family members if care was effective.
   b. Ask a visitor who might be objective if the care he or she observed was effective.
   c. Discuss care in a team conference to evaluate effectiveness.
   d. Ask healthcare providers in community agencies who are in touch with clients after discharge.

3. Michelle Peters has just discovered she has cancer of the lungs. The nurse sits with her and holds her hand as she crys. This action by the nurse represents which kind of skill?
   a. Intellectual
   b. Technical
   c. Interdependent
   d. Interpersonal

37

Documenting and Reporting

Common Acronyms or Terms

APIE	CBE	MIS	RIE
DAPE	MAR	PIE	SOAP
DAR	MDS	RAP	SOAPIER

CHAPTER OVERVIEW

Chapter 37 discusses the health record and various documentation systems. The process of reporting is also discussed. The purpose and content of the health record is also addressed.

✪ Be sure to review the Learning Objectives from the text.

✔ Be sure to FIRST perform Improving Concentration exercises described in the Introduction before proceeding with the next exercise.

Part 1

Indicate the order in which the following major headings are found in the chapter.

1. _____ Content of the Health Record

2. _____ Reporting

3. _____ Documentation Systems

4. _____ Purposes of the Health Record

5. _____ Guidelines for Documentation

Part 2

Complete the following statements by filling in the blanks.

1. Reporting is an oral method of communication that is t_____, p_____, and accurate.

2. Two types of documentation systems listed under that major heading are m_____ and e_____ records.

3. C_____ means a client's right to privacy that healthcare personnel safeguard in both documentation and reporting.

4. Assessment documents r_____ all c_____ information.

Part 3

Fill in the blocks with the letters of the term that matches the term defined below the line.

1. _____
   A manual or electric account of a client's relationship with a healthcare facility

2. _____ system
   Used by a medical information system for storing, processing, and transmitting client data, treatment, and outcomes

3. _____
   Graph or form that records large amounts of information collected at intervals over a period

4. _____
   Standard form used in long-term care and some home care agencies as part of the admitting nursing history

5. _____
   Another form that aids the nursing care team to create an individualized plan of care for every client

6. _____
   Is entered at regular intervals to summarize the client's condition or response to treatment

Part 4

Complete the following statements by filling in the blanks.

1. Three reasons for maintaining a health record are to facilitate _____ among caregivers, to provide evidence of _____, and to facilitate health _____ and _____.

2. In _____ _____ caregivers move from client to client discussing pertinent information.

3. _____-_-_____ reporting is a means of exchanging information between the outgoing and incoming staff on each shift.

4. A paper health record is considered _____, whereas a record housed in a computer system is considered a _____ record.

5. The four general categories of information contained on the health record are _____ documents, plans for _____ and _____, _____ records, and plans for _____ of ____.

Part 5

Indicate if the following action would be appropriate (A) or inappropriate (I).

1. _____ Describe exactly what you observe and document what you see.

2. _____ Use abbreviations and partial sentences to save time and space when charting; (ie, "Client OK while up OOB.")

3. _____ Document medications as you leave the medication area, to avoid forgetting after you leave the client's room.

4. _____ Use direct quotes and enclose client statements with quotation marks when charting.

5. _____ When charting by exception, list only abnormalities or unexpected findings in the progress notes using SOAPIER format.

6. _____ Leave vacant lines in the health record to allow an opportunity to add information later if necessary.

7. _____ If an error is made during charting, use correction fluid and change incorrect information.

8. _____ Introduce the oncoming nurse to the client to build rapport.

Part 6

Match the statement or terms in column I with the related term or abbreviation in column II.

Column I

1. _____ Very thin
2. _____ Tx
3. _____ Occurs *over a long period* (such as cough)
4. _____ OS
5. _____ Dx
6. _____ How long it lasts
7. _____ Bed-wetting
8. _____ aa
9. _____ Feeling of being unsteady, dizzy
10. _____ PC

Column II

a. Left eye

b. Duration

c. Enuresis

d. Cachectic, emaciated

e. Diagnosis

f. Treatment

g. Vertigo

h. After meals

i. Persistent

j. Of each

38

The Health Care Facility Environment

Common Acronyms or Terms

ASU	NICU
CCU	OB
CDU	OPD
CSS	OPS
ECC	OR
ECF	ORTHO
ECG	OT
ED	PACU
EEG	PEDS
EMG	PICU
ENT	PSYCH
GI	PT
GU	REHAB
GYN	RT
ICU	SCU
MRI	SDSU
NEURO	SNF

CHAPTER OVERVIEW

Chapter 38 addresses aspects of the healthcare facility. The client unit, hospital personnel, and services and nursing care are discussed.

✪ Be sure to review the Learning Objectives from the text.

✔ Be sure to FIRST perform Improving Concentration exercises described in the Introduction before proceeding with the next exercise.

Part 1

Indicate if the following headings would be found under The Client Unit (CU), Provision of Nursing Care (PN), or Hospital Personnel and Services (HP).

1. _____ Restocking the Unit

2. _____ Support Services

3. _____ Components of the Basic Client Unit

4. _____ Direct Client Care Departments

5. _____ Diagnostic and Treatment Departments

Part 2

Complete the following statements by filling in the blanks.

1. The _____ is the area in which you deliver most nursing care.

2. Many services provided in the hospital are also provided in ECFs, _____, and the _____.

3. A _____ and _____ unit helps to prevent accidents and infections.

4. In a clinic setting a _____ _____ holds the equipment used in the examination.

5. The _____ is the place where dead bodies are kept.

Part 3

Match the definitions in column I with the terms in column II.

Column I

1. _____ Toilet that is portable, lightweight, and sturdy

2. _____ They determine the underlying nature of diseases through their examination and study of tissue specimen.

3. _____ A place where studies and experiments on animals are conducted

4. _____ In this department radiation therapy and CT scans are done.

5. _____ Also known as the cardiopulmonary department

6. _____ Department uses diversional or craft activities to help clients toward rehabilitation

7. _____ Examinations of a body after death

8. _____ Enables healthcare providers to communicate with clients in different locations using a telephone and computer

Column II

a. Telecommunications

b. Autopsies

c. Respiratory therapy

d. Nuclear medicine

e. Commode

f. Pathologist

g. Research laboratory

h. Occupational therapy

Part 4

Supply the department responsible for the activities provided (abbreviations provide a hint).

1. _____ (CCU)
   Cares for clients with serious heart disorders

2. _____ (PEDS) unit
   Responsible for the care of children

3. _____ (REHAB)
   Provides physical medicine, psychosocial support, and other services to people who have physical disability to help them regain as much capacity for activity as possible

4. _____ _____ (ED)
   Gives care to persons whose conditions require immediate attention

5. _____ (OB)
   Sometimes called the birthing center; provides care to mothers and newborns

6. _____ (also called palliative care)
   Gives physical and emotional care to dying individuals

7. _____ (CSS)
   Cleans and sterilizes equipment for use throughout the hospital

8. _____ (also called continuous quality improvement)
   Promotes the organization's efforts toward quality care

9. _____
   Department responsible for cleaning units in hospitals and ECFs; help prevent the spread of infection

10. _____ (CDU)
    Provides care for persons who abuse chemical substances

Part 5

Complete the following examples of general guidelines for nursing procedures.

1. Follow _ _ _ _ _ _ _ _ Procedures.

2. Wash _ _ _ _ _ _ _ _ _ before and after each procedure.

3. Avoid using the words _ _ _ _ or _ _ _ _ _ _ _ ; say instead "you may feel some discomfort."

4. Make the client as _ _ _ _ _ _ _ _ _ _ as possible before beginning a procedure.

5. Stay with a client during _ _ _ _ _ _ _ _ _ _ _ and procedures.

6. Ask for _ _ _ _ when you need it.

39

Emergency Preparedness

CHAPTER OVERVIEW

Chapter 39 provides an overview of safety procedures in the healthcare facility. Preparation needed for client and employee safety is discussed. The disaster and fire plans are addressed.

✪ Be sure to review the Learning Objectives from the text.

🖎 Be sure to FIRST perform Improving Concentration exercises described in the Introduction before proceeding with the next exercise.

Part 1

Indicate if the following subheadings would be found under the major headings of Safety and Preparedness (SP), the Disaster Plan (DP), or the Fire Plan (FP).

1. _____ Prevention

2. _____ Client Safety

3. _____ Staff Notification

4. _____ General Procedures

5. _____ Emergency Preparedness

Part 2

Complete the following statements by filling in the blanks.

1. Staff members must be able to identify potentially _____ substances and describe what to do if exposed to them.

2. Every staff member in a healthcare facility or community setting must be _____ about fire safety.

3. Nurses not only must _____ accidents but also must know _____ _____ _____ if an accident occurs.

Part 3

Supply the term above the definition provided (the number of letters in the word is provided).

1. _____ (6)
   The process of sorting and classifying victims to determine priority of needs

2. _____

   _____

   _____ (8, 7, 10)
   Provide assistance and support in a disaster to many environments both inside and outside healthcare facilities

3. S.T.A.R.T.—system identifies people who are going to die quickly if they do not receive immediate medical care

   _____ (6) triage and _____

   (5) _____ (9)

4. _____ disaster (8)
   Occurs outside the facility but impairs normal operations

5. _____

   _____ (7, 6)
   In a disaster, it provides overall direction of the facility's activities.

6. _____ disaster (8)
   Occurs when the facility itself is in danger or damaged and function is impaired

7. _____,

   _____,

   _____,

   _____ (6, 5, 7, 10)
   R.A.C.E. Order of procedure a nurse should follow for a fire

8. _____ _____ (8, 4)
   Describes the actions to take in the event of a disaster

Part 4 Completions and Short Answer Exercises

Answer the following questions by filling in the blanks.

1. List five safety tips to remember when using and storing hazardous substances. _____

   _____

2. Potentially hazardous materials include flammables, _____, _____

   _____, _____,

   and harmful physical agents.

3. Complete the following statements regarding accident prevention:

   a. Keep halls free of _____ and promote good order.

   b. Check electrical cords for _____,

      _____ _____,

      and _____.

   c. Get adequate _____ to move and walk clients.

   d. Use _____ _____ for clients who are very old, very young, or disoriented.

   e. Provide adequate _____.

Part 5

Match the class of fire extinguisher in column I with the type of fire used for in column II. Multiple answers apply for many.

Column I

1. _____ Pressurized water

2. _____ Carbon dioxide

3. _____ Dry chemical

4. _____ All purpose

Column II

a. Class A fires: wood, paper, etc.

b. Class B fires: flammable liquids, etc.

c. Class C fires: electrical fires

40

Microbiology and Defense Against Disease

Common Acronyms or Terms

AIDS

ECHO

HIV

MRSA

TB

VRE

CHAPTER OVERVIEW

Chapter 40 discusses microorganisms and infectious disease. A description of microorganisms is provided with detailed overview of the course of infection. Factors that influence infection are addressed.

✪ Be sure to review the Learning Objectives from the text.

✔ Be sure to FIRST perform Improving Concentration exercises described in the Introduction before proceeding with the next exercise.

Part 1

Match the headings in column I with the major headings in this chapter under which they may be found in column II.

Column I

1. _____ Study
2. _____ Actions of Pathogens in the Body
3. _____ Structure and Function
4. _____ Factors That Influence Infection
5. _____ Chain of Infection

Column II

a. Microorganisms

b. Infectious Disease

c. Response to Infection

Part 2

Unscramble the letters, then fill in term or terms that best match(es) the definition.

1. Mucamonbelic _____
   Microorganisms that can spread from one person to another

2. Stocogunia _____
   Diseases that are communicable and are transmitted to many individuals quickly and easily

3. Sysocim _____
   Infection caused by a fungus

4. Trovec _____
   Live carrier of pathogens; include flies, mosquitoes, and fleas as examples

5. Tixonexos _____
   Poisonous substances manufactured by a microorganism and excreted into the surrounding tissue

6. Aspristae _____
   Microorganisms that live on or within another living being (the host)

7. Perastuviup _____
   Pus-forming

8. Xiont _____
   Poison produced by microorganisms

9. Teghopan _____
   Microorganisms that cause disease

10. Luverinec _____
    Pathogen's strength to cause disease

Part 3

Match the concepts in column I with the related terms in column II.

1. _____ Minute living cells not visible to the naked eye; found almost everywhere in the environment

2. _____ Oxygen, nutrients, temperature, moisture, pH, and light

3. _____ Physical shape, movement, Gram's stain reaction, and relationship to oxygen

4. _____ Microorganisms that do not usually cause disease, but can do so if person is susceptible

5. _____ Time from when the pathogen enters the body to the appearance of the first symptoms of illness

6. _____ The period from the onset of initial symptoms (such as fatigue) to more severe symptoms

Column II

a. Opportunistic microorganisms

b. Prodromal stage

c. Ways in which bacteria are classified

d. Microorganisms

e. Factors that influence microorganism growth

f. Incubation period

Part 4 Short Answer Exercises

Complete these short answer questions by filling in the blanks.

1. Factors that influence whether or not disease-causing microorganisms will cause an infection include specific _____ of _____, number of _____, _____, and host _____.

2. Describe the five main types of microorganisms and the basic characteristics of each.

   _____

3. Discuss ways to prevent the development of drug-resistant bacteria.

   _____

Part 5

Organize the following points in the chain of infection to indicate how infection is spread.

1. Portal(s) of entry
2. Exit from reservoir
3. Susceptible host
4. Reservoir for growth and reproduction of infectious agents
5. Vehicles of transmission

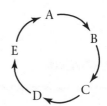

41

Nosocomial Infections and Medical Asepsis

Common Acronyms or Terms

CDC   PPE

CHAPTER OVERVIEW

Chapter 41 discusses infection and techniques needed to prevent the spread of infection in healthcare facility. The implications of nosocomial infections for the client and nurse are addressed. The concept of medical asepsis and use of antimicrobial agents to prevent the spread of infection are addressed.

✪ Be sure to review the Learning Objectives from the text.

✔ Be sure to FIRST perform Improving Concentration exercises described in the Introduction before proceeding with the next exercise.

Part 1

Indicate the order in which the following major headings and subheadings are found in the chapter.

1. _____ Client and Family Teaching
2. _____ Clients and Nosocomial Infections
3. _____ Medical Asepsis
4. _____ Barrier Techniques
5. _____ Handwashing

Part 2

Complete the following statements by filling in the blanks.

1. _____ infections are acquired in healthcare facilities.
2. Commonly used protective barriers include _____, eye protection, _____ and _____.
3. Teaching _____ practices to clients, families, and visitors is essential to protection against disease.
4. Barrier techniques are located under the major heading of _____ _____.

Part 3

Fill in the blocks with the letters of the term that matches the definition below the line.

1. _
   Used to keep organisms from entering or leaving the respiratory tract (yours or the client's); examples include gloves and eye protection

2. _ _ _ _ _ _ _ _ _ _ _ _ _
   Refers to the practice of reducing the number of microorganisms or preventing and reducing transmission of microorganisms from one person (or source) to another

3. _
   Chemicals that decrease the number of pathogens in an area

4. _ _ _ _ _ _ _ _
   Therapy that enters the body by a means other than normal; includes surgery, tracheotomies as examples

5. _ _ _ _ _ _ _ _ _ _
   Organisms that are present within the person's body

6. _ _ _ _ _ _ _ _ _ _
   Blood infections; one of the most common nosocomial infections

Part 4

Complete the following statements or short answer exercises by filling in the blanks.

1. Three components of medical asepsis include reducing the number of skin microorganisms through _____ (the best method of disease prevention); use of _____ techniques (eg, gowns, gloves); and keeping the environment _____ and _____ to reduce disease transmission.

2. The Centers for Disease Control and Prevention (CDC) recommend routine handwashing for a duration of _____ to _____ seconds and for _____ if your hands are visibly soiled.

3. A person's risk for developing a nosocomial infection increases when certain conditions exist. Name three such conditions.

   _____

   _____

   _____

4. Barrier techniques include using a _____ when giving care to a client with a communicable disease that is transmitted through the respiratory tract, using _____ protection if any danger exists of a client's body fluids splashing or spraying onto you, and using _____ when you must touch blood or body fluids.

5. The nurse can play a role in preventing nosocomial infections by breaking the chain of infection. The nurse should minimize the _____ and _____ of organism spread to potential infection sites, control portals of _____ and _____, avoid actions that _____ microorganisms, and prevent bacteria from finding a _____ to _____.

Part 5

Indicate if the following action would be appropriate (A) or inappropriate (I).

1. _____ Removing soiled gloves by grasping the inside of one glove first and pulling it off, then grasping the inside of the other glove and pulling it off with the first glove inside.

2. _____ Using double-bag technique to remove contaminated refuse and linen from a client's room

3. _____ Shaking linen to remove loose debris, then placing it on the floor for removal when fresh linen is on the bed

4. _____ Sending items to be sterilized to central supply room in plastic bags

5. _____ Monitoring the compliance of others regarding infection control practices

6. _____ Using nonprescribed medications only if they belong to other family members who had similar symptoms

7. _____ Removing jewelry, except a plain wedding band, before washing hands

8. _____ When washing hands, wetting your hands and forearms with water, keeping the hands lower than your elbows

42

Infection Control

Common Acronyms or Terms

BBP

CDC

HICPAC

IV

TB

CHAPTER OVERVIEW

Chapter 42 discusses the precautions taken for control of the spread of infection. Isolation and barrier techniques are addressed.

✪ Be sure to review the Learning Objectives from the text.

❦ Be sure to FIRST perform Improving Concentration exercises described in the Introduction before proceeding with the next exercise.

Part 1

Complete the following titles or statements related to major headings and key points in this chapter.

1. The first major heading is Infection C _ _ _ _ _ _ .

2. Special filtered r _ _ _ _ _ _ _ _ _ m_ _ _ _ are required when caring for a client with known or suspected TB.

3. P _ _ _ _ _ _ _ _ isolation prevents organisms from coming into contact with clients.

4. B_ _ _ _ _ _ techniques prevent microorganisms from leaving a client's room.

5. The last major heading in the chapter is The Infection C_ _ _ _ _ _ C_ _ _ _ _ _ _ .

Part 2 Key Terms: Knowledge Check

Match the key terms with the appropriate definition.

Column I

1. _____ Airborne Precautions

2. _____ Contact Precautions

3. _____ Droplet Precautions

4. _____ Transmission-based Precautions

5. _____ Standard Precautions

Column II

a. Designed for clients with specific infections or diagnoses

b. Needed when droplets containing microorganisms are propelled through the air from an infected person and deposited on the host's eyes, nose, or mouth

c. Designed for the care of all clients regardless of diagnosis or infection status; a combination of Universal Precautions and Body Substance Isolation

d. Needed when tiny microorganisms from evaporated droplets remain suspended in the air or are carried on dust particles and a susceptible host can easily inhale the microorganisms

e. Required when disease transmission can occur through direct touch between a susceptible host's body surface and an infected person or intermediate contaminated object

Part 3

Fill in the term or terms that best complete(s) the statement.

1. _____ occurs when a microorganism is present in a client but she shows no clinical signs or symptoms of infection.

2. Standard Precautions apply to all body fluids, secretions, and excretions except _____, nonintact _____, and _____ membranes.

3. Standard Precautions require that you change gloves after each _____ with a client.

4. Wear a _____, _____, _____, and _____ if splashing or spraying of blood or body fluids is possible.

5. When feeding a client the nurse should perform _____ and wear _____ to decrease blood-borne pathogen exposure.

6. When handling lab specimens the nurse should perform _____ and wear _____, and use _____, _____, and _____ if splattering is likely.

7. When setting up a client's room for isolation, the bedside _____ or cabinet stocked with _____ as required for the client's condition should be left outside the room or in an anteroom.

8. While administering medications the nurse should use _____ medication cups and if a medication tray is used, it should be _____.

Part 4

Indicate the barrier precautions needed by marking the statement with Gl for gloves, G for gown, M for mask on nurse, MC for mask on client, H for handwashing, E for eyewear, N for none. Multiple letters are often required.

1. _____ Airborne precautions—entering the room to look at a bedside monitor

2. _____ Examining a client's mouth, teeth, and gums

3. _____ Performing an operative procedure with high possibility of blood splashing

4. _____ Talking with a client who is not on transmission-based precautions

5. _____ Transporting a client who is on droplet precautions

43

Emergency Care and Sudden Death

Common Acronyms or Terms

ABCDE   LOC

ACLS   MAST

AED   MUA

AVPU   PERRLA+C

BLS, BCLS   RICE

CNS   SIDS

CPR   SIRES

ED   SubQ

EMS

CHAPTER OVERVIEW

Chapter 43 addresses the principles of emergency care. The occurrence of sudden death and life support are also discussed. An overview of advanced cardiac life support and the concept of and steps included in basic cardiac life support is provided.

✪ Be sure to review the Learning Objectives from the text.

✔ Be sure to FIRST perform Improving Concentration exercises described in the Introduction before proceeding with the next exercise.

Part 1

Complete the following titles and statements found as major headings and key points in this chapter.

1. Basic cardiac life support and advanced cardiac life support are discussed under which major heading in this chapter? _____ _____ and _____ _____

2. The heading Two-Rescuer CPR contains two sub-heading titles: When CPR is in _____ and When CPR _____ _____ in _____.

3. Nurses must use _____ _____ when giving first aid to whatever extent possible.

4. Calling _____ will summon the EMS system in almost all areas of the United States and Canada.

5. Be sure to treat an injured person for _____.

Part 2 Key Terms: Knowledge Check

Review the key terms in the chapter. Mark (y) beside the terms you know the definition of and (n) beside the terms you do not know. List the terms marked with an (n) in the spaces below and write the definition of each as you read.

Term

_____

_____

_____

_____

Definition

_____

_____

_____

_____

_____

_____

Part 3 Matching of Key Terms: Knowledge Check

Match the following key terms in the chapter with the appropriate definition.

Column I

1. _____ Abdominal thrusts
2. _____ Anaphylaxis
3. _____ Antidote
4. _____ Cafe coronary
5. _____ Caustic
6. _____ Intubation
7. _____ Mediastinal shift
8. _____ Recovery position
9. _____ Rescue breathing
10. _____ Tourniquet

Column II

a. Inserting a tube into the person's trachea

b. Oxygen from the rescuer inflates the victim's lungs

c. Roll the person onto the side, moving the head, shoulders, and torso simultaneously without twisting them

d. When the heart, great vessels, and the tracheal move over to the side opposite the injury; may occur when a tension pneumothorax remains uncorrected

e. Another name for the Heimlich maneuver; may perform on an adult or child

f. A person who has an airway obstruction (choking) goes off alone and is found not breathing and without a pulse (an apparent heart attack victim)

g. A tie used on an extremity over a pressure point to stop hemorrhage

h. A type I allergic, life-threatening reaction to a substance

i. A substance that neutralizes poisons

j. Substances that are extremely irritating

Part 4

Indicate if the following actions would be appropriate (A) or inappropriate (I) in emergencies.

1. _____ Do not move any injured person if you assess that the area is safe.

2. _____ Assist in an emergency only to the level of your first aid training.

3. _____ Monitor for falling blood pressure and unresponsiveness as early signs of shock.

4. _____ Administer high concentrations of oxygen, if available, when treating shock in an emergency.

5. _____ Tape a dressing on all four sides over a puncture chest wound to prevent air from entering the chest.

6. _____ Always treat the victim of an MVA or fall as though he or she has a back or neck injury.

7. _____ Keep a potential head injury victim lying flat and restricting his or her movements.

8. _____ Place frostbitten body parts in water that is between 98° and 104°F.

9. _____ Give a person who is experiencing heat cramps a glass of water and two salt tablets.

10. _____ Apply indirect pressure to the wound and lower the injured part to stop bleeding.

Part 5

Complete the following statements by filling in the blanks.

1. _____ death occurs when a person's breathing and heartbeat stop, while _____ death refers to permanent damage of brain cells due to lack of oxygen; _____ death is irreversible.

2. _____ death occurs any time breathing and the heartbeat stop abruptly or unexpectedly.

3. The _____ _____ _____ is considered the definitive initial treatment of victims in cardiac arrest.

4. The letters A,B,C,D,E represent the order for assessing the person in an emergency and represent: Airway and cervical spine, B _____, C _____ and _____, D _____, E _____ and _____.

5. A person experiencing heat _____ demonstrates cool skin with normal or below normal body temperature, whereas a person with Heat _____ exhibits hot skin with a high temperature.

6. The acronym RICE in emergency procedures for sprains and strains means:
R _____, I _____,
C _____, and E _____.

Part 6

Indicate the correct order for the following steps in cardiopulmonary resuscitation.

1. _____ Open the airway
2. _____ Perform external chest compressions
3. _____ Position the person
4. _____ Determine breathlessness
5. _____ Activate the EMS system
6. _____ Check the pulse
7. _____ Determine unresponsiveness
8. _____ Perform rescue breathing if the heart is beating

44

Therapeutic Communication Skills

CHAPTER OVERVIEW

Chapter 44 focuses on the importance of effective communication as part of the nursing process.

✪ Be sure to review the Learning Objectives from the text.

✔ Be sure to FIRST perform Improving Concentration exercises described in the Introduction before proceeding with the next exercise.

Part 1

Match the subheadings in column I with the major headings in column II.

Column I

1. _____ Types of Communication
2. _____ Physician's Orders
3. _____ Interviewing
4. _____ Communicating in Special Situations
5. _____ Factors Influencing Communication

Column II

a. Communication

b. Therapeutic Communication Techniques

c. Communications Among the Healthcare Team

Part 2

Answer these statements true (T) or false (F). Correct the false.

1. _____ An interview is a non–goal-directed conversation in which one person seeks information from the other.

2. _____ Verbal communication can be written or spoken.

3. _____ Aphasia is the ability to communicate verbally.

4. _____ Personal space usually extends outward from the body about 1.5 to 2 feet.

5. _____ Nonverbal communication is also called body language.

Part 3 Critical Thinking

You are the student nurse taking care of Mrs. Evans and you have just finished taking her vital signs and bathing her, when her family doctor comes in, talks to her briefly and says to you. "Her output is down, I want you to give her another 30 mg of Lasix this morning." As a student nurse, how do you respond?

_____

_____

Part 4

Complete the sentences by filling in the blanks.

1. _____ and _____ are two factors that can influence communication.

2. Verbal _____ are designed to stop the communication process.

3. _____ _____ means looking directly to the eyes of another person.

4. Physician's orders tell the nurse what to do, nursing _____ show how to do it.

5. Communication requires several components, which include sender, _____, channel _____, and interaction.

45

Admission, Transfer, and Discharge

CHAPTER OVERVIEW

Chapter 45 outlines the different components of client care involved in the admission, transfer, and discharge process.

✪ Be sure to review the Learning Objectives from the text.

✔ Be sure to FIRST perform Improving Concentration exercises described in the Introduction before proceeding with the next exercise.

Part 1

Indicate the order in which the following major headings are found in the chapter.

_____ Discharge

_____ Admission

_____ Leaving the Healthcare Facility Against Advice

_____ Transfer to Another Unit

Part 2 Multiple Choice

Circle the letter corresponding to the correct answer.

1. Advance directives:
   a. Allow the family to specify choices of healthcare treatment without client input
   b. Are only to provide information about healthcare choices
   c. Are required by law to be discussed on admission to healthcare facilities
   d. Are verbal agreements allowing an individual to specify healthcare choices

2. A sling-type apparatus that looks like a suspended hammock used to weigh immobile patients is called a:
   a. Chair scale
   b. Litter scale
   c. Balance scale
   d. Digital scale

3. On admission the client's bed should be:
   a. In the high position
   B. In the low position
   C. At the mid-point
   D. In semi-Fowler's position

4. Vital signs do not routinely include:
   a. Temperature
   b. Pulse
   c. Pulse pressure
   d. Blood pressure

5. Discharge teaching is individual and:
   ?. Insight oriented
   b. Assessment motivated
   c. Goal-directed
   d. Must be documented

6. Discharge planning begins:
   a. On admission
   b. After orientation to the floor/unit
   c. After transfer from one unit to another
   d. On the last hospital day

Part 3

Indicate whether the actions described below are part of admission (A), transfer (T), or discharge (D).

1. _____ Determine how the client will be moved.

2. _____ Teach the client the proper operation of equipment and care of tubes.

3. _____ Provide information about public health and home nursing services.

4. _____ Assemble all the client's personal belongings, double check for all clothes and other articles.

5. _____ Be sure the client receives and wears an identification band.

Part 4

Complete the sentences by filling in the blanks.

1. The healthcare facility assumes _____ _____ for articles left at the bedside.

2. Weigh the client on admission and _____ or weekly before the client eats.

3. When a child is ill, _____ often occurs.

4. _____ may cause physical and emotional stress that can aggravate a client's health problem.

5. It is important that each client receive an _____ _____. Check the information on it to see that it is correct.

6. _____ is the process of depriving a person of personality, spirit, and other human qualities.

Part 5 Clinical Thinking

You are preparing Miguel Mendoza for discharge. Discuss at least five of the general discharge instructions you will discuss with him. Use the chart on page 493 in your textbook.

_____

_____

_____

_____

_____

_____

46

Vital Signs

Common Acronyms or Terms

Ap	HR
A-R	I & O
Ax	MAP
BP	PO
BPM	R, PR
C	SBP
DBP	TPR
F	VS

CHAPTER OVERVIEW

Chapter 46 discusses the measurements that are indicators of the functions necessary to sustain life.

✪ Be sure to review the Learning Objectives from the text.

✔ Be sure to FIRST perform Improving Concentration exercises described in the Introduction before proceeding with the next exercise.

Part 1

Complete the following statements related to the headings and key points in the chapter.

1. The first major heading addresses "The _____ _____."

2. The remaining major headings discuss assessing body temperature, _____, _____, and _____, and _____.

3. Documentation of vital signs is essential to _____ _____ regarding the client's status and _____ _____ _____.

4. _____ is the vibration of the blood through the arteries as the heart beats. It is measured by rate and rhythm.

5. _____ is the process by which the lungs bring oxygen into the body and remove carbon dioxide.

Part 2 Multiple Choice

Circle the letter corresponding to the correct answer.

1. Blood pressure is a measurement of the pressure the blood exerts on:
   a. Walls of veins
   b. Walls of capillaries
   c. Walls of arteries
   d. Walls of organs

2. The most accurate pulse, especially for children under age 2 years, is the:
   a. Apical
   b. Radial
   c. Carotid
   d. Popliteal

3. The correct term to describe a sudden drop from fever to normal temperature is:
   a. Remittent
   b. Intermittent
   c. Lysis
   d. Crises

4. Abnormally slow breathing, below 10/minute is documented as:
   a. Eupnea
   b. Bradypnea
   c. Apnea
   d. Tachypnea

5. Measurement of blood pressure with a sphygmomanometer is considered:
   a. Mercury
   b. Aneroid
   c. Direct
   d. Indirect

Part 3 Clinical Thinking

Mr. Charles Hampton, a 64-year-old schoolteacher, has vital signs as follows:

Temperature 98.8

Pulse 78

Respirations 18

Blood pressure 190/100

Using this information answer the following questions.

1. Are all his vital signs within normal limits? If not, document the abnormal and state the normal value(s).
2. What is Mr. Hampton's MAP?
3. What site were you most likely to use to determine body temperature? Why?
4. What words would you use to describe his pulse rhythm?
5. What medical term describes Mr. Hampton's breathing rate?

Part 4 True or False

Answer these statements true (T) or false (F). Correct the false.

1. _____ Oral and rectal thermometers can be used interchangeably.

2. _____ Normal body temperature is approximately 37° Celsius.

3. _____ Clinical hypothermia is life-threatening and requires immediate treatment.

4. _____ The diaphragm of a stethoscope is used to hear breath sounds, normal heartbeat, and bowel signs.

5. _____ Cheyne-Stokes respirations are slow and shallow at first, but grow gradually faster and deeper.

47

Assessment and Physical Examination

Common Acronyms or Terms

CO_2

CT

ECG

EEG

LOC

LP

MRI

O_2

PET

PMI

CHAPTER OVERVIEW

Chapter 47 addresses the process of assessment and physical examination by the nurse. An overview of the course of disease and common risk factors for disease and illness is provided. Physical examination techniques and common tests and procedures that healthcare providers use are also discussed.

✪ Be sure to review the Learning Objectives from the text.

✔ Be sure to FIRST perform Improving Concentration exercises described in the Introduction before proceeding with the next exercise.

Part 1

Complete the following titles and statements found as major headings and key points in this chapter.

1. The course of the disease and the body's response to disease are found under which major heading in this chapter: F _ _ _ _ _ _ that I _ _ _ _ _ _ _ _ A _ _ _ _ _ _ _ _ _.

2. The heading Medical Diagnosis contains subheadings that include: Special Diagnostic Procedures and L _ _ _ _ _ _ _ _ _ T _ _ _ _.

3. D _____ is a change in body structure. I _____ is the individual's response to change in function.

4. Diseases are categorized in many ways according to _____ or the _____ on the person.

5. The most common formats for the physical examination are the ___-__-___ examination or the examination done by _____ _____.

Part 2 Matching of Key Terms: Knowledge Check

Match the following key terms in the chapter with the appropriate definition.

Column I

1. _____ Smegma
2. _____ Symptom
3. _____ Wheal
4. _____ Vesicle
5. _____ Lordosis
6. _____ Secondary disease
7. _____ Malaise
8. _____ Herniation
9. _____ Complication
10. _____ Induration

Column II

a. Hardened tissue

b. Generalized discomfort

c. An unexpected event in the disease course that often delays the client's recovery

d. Subjective evidence of disease, sensations that only the client knows and can report

e. Lesion slightly irregular in shape; transient superficial elevated area of localized edema

f. Physical wasting of tissues

g. Cheesy substance; accumulates under the foreskin of the penis

h. Small skin lesion, well-defined border; elevated cavity filled with serous fluid

i. Directly results or depends on another disorder

j. Outpouching of tissue; appears around the umbilicus at the inguinal line or around incisions

Part 3

Most of the following statements are incorrect. Correct the following statements, if needed, by substituting the correct term for the incorrect term.

1. _____ A *bronchoscopy* estimates the percentage of oxygenated blood flow through a body part.

2. _____ *Auscultation* is feeling body tissues or parts with your hands or fingers.

3. _____ The *patch or scratch test* identifies tissue abnormalities.

4. _____ *Cardiac catheterization* measures pressures within heart chambers to determine muscle strength, valve function, cardiac output, and fluid volume.

5. _____ *Cholangiography* allows direct visualization of the esophagus, stomach, and duodenum.

6. _____ *Percussion* is careful, close, and detailed visual examination of a body part.

7. _____ The *echocardiogram* graphically records the electrical impulses of cardiac musculature to identify dysrhythmias or tissue damage.

8. _____ *Endoscopy* allows visualization of body tissues through a series of images recorded in layers.

Part 4 Multiple Choice

Circle the letter corresponding to the correct answer.

1. Mila Pollin returns to your floor after having a cholecystogram. She complains of her nose itching and states she feels cold. The nurse should explain that:
   a. The cholecystogram causes a chronic inflammation and the itching results from generalized chronic effects and the cold sensation from the localized effects.
   b. She should expect such symptoms because the tube was inserted into her nose so a diagnosis could be made.
   c. The symptoms could be signs of an allergic reaction to the dye used in the test so the physician will be notified immediately.
   d. The sneezing and cold sensation will soon disappear because they resulted from the cold temperature in the lab where she took the test and extra blankets will help.

2. When beginning to perform a physical examination, the nurse should explain the purpose of the examination and close the door to the room or draw curtains around the bedside. In addition, the nurse should:
   a. Ask the client to empty the bladder or bowel if necessary.
   b. Tell the client to soak in a tub of water to reduce skin organisms the nurse might contact.
   c. Have the client examine his or her perineal area and describe observations to avoid embarrassment.
   d. Administer a sedative so the client will be relaxed and extremities can be moved as needed.

3. When performing a skin assessment, which of the following would be cause for concern?
   a. Mucous membranes and nailbeds in an African American client are pink to dark pink.
   b. Skin on the hand feels plump, firm, and elastic; skin is slightly moist.
   c. Skin temperature is warm to touch with head and trunk warmer than feet and hands.
   d. Extremities are cool and pale in color with swelling over the bony prominences.

4. You suspect Michel Aguiela has problems with his musculoskeletal function. Which of the following data might support your suspicion?
   a. Abnormal breath sounds are noted, including rales and wheezes.
   b. Both legs are weak and the client is unable to push against force.
   c. Pulse is irregular with an intensity difference between the carotid and apical pulses.
   d. Client reports abdominal tenderness or pain and shows guarding and rigidity.

48

Body Mechanics

Common Acronyms or Terms

AROM	PROM
CPM	ROM
OOB	

CHAPTER OVERVIEW

Chapter 48 addresses the principles of proper body mechanics and the use of these mechanics in the positioning and mobility of clients. The safety of the nurse and client is discussed. An overview of mobility and safety devices is provided.

✪ Be sure to review the Learning Objectives from the text.

✔ Be sure to FIRST perform Improving Concentration exercises described in the Introduction before proceeding with the next exercise.

Part 1

Complete the following titles and statements found as major headings and key points in this chapter.

1. The final major heading in this chapter is P_ _ _ _ _

    _ _ _ _ _ for E_ _ _ _ _ _ _ _ _ _

2. The major heading Body Mechanics in Client Positioning contains subheadings that include: Assisting the Mobile Client, Using Mobility Devices,

Using S_ _ _ _ _ Devices, Moving Clients Who Are P_ _ _ _ _ _ _, and Using the Wheeled Stretcher.

3. P _ _ _ _ _ _, pushing or r_ _ _ _ _ an object is easier than is lifting it. It usually requires less energy or force to keep an object moving than to s_ _ _ _ and s _ _ _ it.

4. A client may become d_ _ _ _ or faint whenever you first help him or her out of bed.

Part 2 Matching of Key Terms: Knowledge Check

Match the following key terms in the chapter with the appropriate definition.

Column I

1. _____ Abduction
2. _____ Adduction
3. _____ Hemiplegia
4. _____ Eversion
5. _____ Extension
6. _____ Flexion
7. _____ Paraplegic
8. _____ Range of motion
9. _____ Supination
10. _____ Contractures

Column II

a. Turning the foot so the sole faces away from the other foot

b. Increasing the angle between two bones

c. Turning the foot so its sole faces the other foot; inversion

d. Moving a part toward the body's midline

e. Decreasing the angle between two bones

f. The continuous contraction (shortening of the length) of the muscles that move the bones of the joint

g. A person who is paralyzed from the waist area down

h. Paralysis occurring on one side of the body

i. Each body joint's specific but limited opening and closing motion

j. Moving a part away from the midline of the body

Part 3

Indicate if the following actions would be appropriate (A) or Inappropriate (I).

1. _____ When logroll turning the client, keep the body in a straight alignment.

2. _____ Place a client in a protective prone position with head turned sideways for long periods to prevent aspiration and minimize headache.

3. _____ Use pillows to support the head, neck, arms, and hands when a client is lying on the back.

4. _____ In a modified Sims' position (alternative side-lying) you ask the client to keep knees straight.

5. _____ When moving an immobile client to the side of the bed, bend at the back and pull with your arms.

6. _____ Use a transfer board or bridge for clients who are unable to stand.

Part 4

Complete the following short answer or fill-in-the blank exercises.

1. What are two of the principles underlying proper body mechanics? _____

_____

_____

_____

_____

2. When assisting clients out of bed, the nurse should assume a _____ base of support.

3. A person's center of gravity is located in the _____ area.

4. Stretching the body as tall as you can produces proper body _____.

5. If you draw an imaginary vertical line through the top of your head, center of gravity, and base of support you have determined your line of gravity or _____ plane.

Part 5

Organize the following steps in dangling the bedridden client:

1. _____ Roll a pillow and tuck it firmly behind the client's back.

2. _____ Place one arm around the client's shoulders and your other arm under his or her knees.

3. _____ Measure and record the client's pulse and blood pressure for baseline.

4. _____ After some time, help the client lie down again by supporting his or her shoulders and knees and turning him or her back around.

5. _____ Document the procedure.

6. _____ Dangle the client's legs for as long as ordered if tolerated.

7. _____ Elevate the head of the bed as high as it will go.

8. _____ Turn the client toward you so his or her feet touch the floor.

49

Beds and Bedmaking

CHAPTER OVERVIEW

Chapter 49 discusses the process of bed making. The different stages of bed making and types of equipment used with beds for clients who are ill are addressed.

✪ Be sure to review the Learning Objectives from the text.

✔ Be sure to FIRST perform Improving Concentration exercises described in the Introduction before proceeding with the next exercise.

Part 1

Complete the following titles and statements found as major headings and key points in this chapter.

1. The final major heading in this chapter is _____ Beds and _____.

2. The major heading Attachments and Accessories contains subheadings that include: Bed _____, Side _____, and Other _____.

3. Organize _____. Gather all supplies _____ making the bed. Strip and make _____ side of the bed at a time to conserve _____ and _____.

4. Place _____ linen in a pillow case or on a _____ while continuing your work.

Part 2 Matching of Key Terms: Knowledge Check

Match the following key terms in the chapter with the appropriate definition.

Column I

1. _____ Bed cradle
2. _____ Closed bed
3. _____ Egg crate mattress
4. _____ Mitered
5. _____ Open bed

Column II

a. Foam rubber and shaped like an egg carton

b. A diagonal corner used for tucking sheets that are not fitted

c. A frame used to prevent the bedclothes from touching all or part of the client's body

d. Used when preparing the unit for a new client; also called unoccupied beds

e. Allow linens to be turned down, making it easier for the client to get into bed

Part 3

Indicate if the following actions would be appropriate (A) or inappropriate (I).

1. _____ Preparing an open bed for a client returning from the operating room or another procedure

2. _____ Fanfolding the top bedding down to the foot of the mattress when making a closed bed

3. _____ Changing bed linens with the client in the bed if client has generalized weakness

4. _____ Using a footboard on the bed to prevent a deformity called footdrop

5. _____ Placing a trapeze over the bed to support the body in correct alignment

6. _____ Using a transfer board or bridge for clients who are unable to stand

Part 4

Indicate if the following steps are appropriate for making an occupied bed (O), closed bed (C), or a postoperative bed (P).

1. _____ Fanfold top linens to the foot of the bed or put top linens over the foundation but do not tuck.

2. _____ Loosen bottom bed linens, fanfold soiled linens from the side of the bed and wedge them close to the client.

3. _____ Tuck in the bottom linens, then pull covers up to the top of the bed.

Part 5

Organize the following steps of preparing an occupied bed.

1. _____ Place the clean bottom bed sheet on the bed folded lengthwise with the center fold as close to the client's back as possible.

2. _____ Place a bath blanket over the top sheet and ask the client to hold it onto the upper edge.

3. _____ Remove the soiled bottom linens.

4. _____ Adjust the bed to a comfortable height, remove the call bell if it is attached to the linens.

5. _____ Loosen bottom bed linens, fanfold soiled linens from the side of the bed, and wedge them close to the client.

6. _____ Grasp clean linens and gently pull them out from under the client, and spread them over the bed's unmade side.

Part 6

Complete the following sentences by filling in the blanks.

1. Side rails _____ clients from falling out of bed and are _____ devices for changing position while clients are in bed.

2. Name two client conditions that might require the use of a bed cradle. _____

3. A bed board may be placed under the mattress to _____ the body in _____ _____.

4. Therapeutic beds are used to treat clients with severe joint _____, prolonged _____, or skin _____ such as burns or pressure ulcers.

5. Therapeutic beds reduce or relieve the effects of _____ against the skin through various mechanisms.

50

Personal Hygiene and Skin Care

CHAPTER OVERVIEW

Chapter 50 addresses the importance of assisting clients who cannot meet their hygiene needs. The skills related to providing basic hygiene and skin care are addressed.

✪ Be sure to review the Learning Objectives from the text.

✔ Be sure to FIRST perform Improving Concentration exercises described in the Introduction before proceeding with the next exercise.

Part 1

Complete the following titles and statements found as major headings and key points in this chapter.

1. The two major headings in this chapter without subheadings are: _____
_____ _____
and _____ _____.

2. The major heading Grooming contains subheadings that include: Caring for _____,
Caring for _____, and
_____ a Client.

3. Encourage the client to provide as _____ personal hygiene and

_____ _____
as possible.

4. The _____ relaxes the client and provides an opportunity for you to observe the client's _____.

Part 2 Matching of Key Terms: Knowledge Check

Match the following key terms in the chapter with the appropriate definition.

Column I

1. _____ Sordes
2. _____ Cerumen
3. _____ Pyorrhea
4. _____ Nits
5. _____ Pediculosis

Column II

a. The eggs of lice; they look like dandruff but are solid specks, not flakes

b. Caused by lice, tiny insects that suck blood from the person they infect

c. Inflammation of the tooth sockets

d. Brownish material that may collect on a client's teeth and tongue with some illnesses

e. Ear wax

Part 3

Indicate if the following actions would be appropriate (A) or inappropriate (I).

1. _____ Offer the client the opportunity to brush his or her teeth before and after each meal and in the morning and evening.

2. _____ When providing mouth care, wear gloves and assist the client to an upright position with an emesis basin in hand.

3. _____ Keep dentures dry in a clean cloth, when the client leaves the dentures out of the mouth.

4. _____ Encourage the client to wear the dentures at all times to prevent gum line changes.

5. _____ When providing mouth care open the client's mouth and insert a padded tongue blade to keep the mouth open.

6. _____ When giving routine eye care, soak cotton balls or gauze squares in peroxide or alcohol.

7. _____ Special eye care for the client who cannot blink includes keeping the eye and surrounding area dry to prevent cross-infection.

8. _____ Wipe the client's eyelid from the inner to the outer canthus to prevent infection.

9. _____ Remove ear wax with a moist Q-Tip and warm saline.

10. _____ Use scissors to cut the client's nails if they are torn or jagged.

Part 4

Complete the following short answer or fill-in-the blank exercises.

1. List three reasons mouth care is particularly valuable to the ill person. _____

2. State three types of cleansing baths and when each one is used. _____

3. Cut toe nails _____ _____ and do not round off the corners.

4. Do not allow a client with _____ hands or poor _____ to shave himself with a blade razor.

5. When braiding hair, start braids toward the _____ for client comfort and safety.

Part 5

Organize the following steps in giving a bed bath.

1. _____ Put the towel over the client's chest and fold the bath blanket back, wash, rinse and dry the client's chest.

2. _____ Raise the bed to a comfortable height for you.

3. _____ Fill the basin about two-thirds full with warm water and place it on the bedside table.

4. _____ Close the curtain or the door.

5. _____ Uncover the client's far leg; wash, rinse and dry it.

6. _____ Lower the side rails and assist the client to turn away from you onto the side; uncover the back and buttocks; wash rinse and dry this area.

7. _____ Provide the client an opportunity to use a bedpan.

8. _____ Give a backrub at this time; tie or snap the client's gown at the back of the neck.

9. _____ Keeping the towel over the client's chest, lower the bath blanket just above the pubic area and wash, rinse and dry the abdomen.

10. _____ Moisten the mitt with plain water and wash the client's eyes.

11. _____ Place the basin on a folded bath towel and immerse the client's foot in water; wash, rinse and dry each foot (immerse one at a time).

12. _____ Change the bath water at this point.

51

Elimination

CHAPTER OVERVIEW

Chapter 51 discusses the process of elimination. Urinary and bowel elimination are addressed. Nursing actions used to assist the client with toileting, urinary elimination, and bowel elimination are discussed.

✪ Be sure to review the Learning Objectives from the text.

✔ Be sure to FIRST perform Improving Concentration exercises described in the Introduction before proceeding with the next exercise.

Part 1

Match the headings in column I with the major headings in this chapter under which they may be found in column II.

Column I

1. _____ The Urinary Catheter
2. _____ Enemas
3. _____ Flatus
4. _____ Bowel Elimination
5. _____ Giving and Removing a Bedpan or Urinal
6. _____ Urinary Retention

Column II

a. Assessing Elimination Function
b. Assisting With Toileting

c. Assisting With Urinary Elimination
d. Assisting With Bowel Elimination

Part 2

Complete the following statements by filling in the blanks.

1. _____ may be a symptom of impacted stool.

2. Assist a client to as _____ a position as possible for elimination and allow for _____.

3. Adequate _____ is a basic function critical to _____.

Part 3

Fill in the term or terms that best match(es) the definition.

1. _____
   Excretion of feces

2. _____
   Decrease in the expected amount of urine a person excretes, usually below 30 mL in 1 hour

3. _____
   Voiding during the night; sometimes occurs when the person drinks a large amount of liquid before bedtime

4. _____
   Painful or burning sensation when passing urine

5. _____
   Inability to empty the bladder of urine

6. _____
   Absence of urine excreted by the kidneys; a sign that the kidneys are functioning improperly

Part 4

Match the following terms in column I with their definitions listed in column II.

Column I

1. _____ Calculi
2. _____ Crede's maneuver

3. _____ Peristalsis

4. _____ Flatus

5. _____ Renal colic

6. _____ Melena

7. _____ Cystitis

8. _____ Incontinence

Column II

a. The application of firm, gentle pressure to the bladder, with hands held flat, starting at the umbilicus and moving down to the symphysis pubis

b. Dark, black, or tarry stool; indicates the presence of digested blood

c. Kidney or bladder stones that develop within the urinary system

d. Infection of the bladder

e. Involuntary loss of urine from the bladder

f. Intestinal gas

g. Muscular action of the intestinal wall that moves feces through the colon

h. Severe penetrating pain in the lower back; may be caused by calculi

Part 5 Short Answer Exercises

Complete the following short answer questions.

1. Briefly discuss the normal characteristics or urine.

   _____

   _____

   _____

2. Two other terms for urination are _____ and _____.

3. Identify the possible causes for common changes in the appearance, consistency, or odor of feces.

   _____

4. Another term for bowel movement or stool is

   _____

5. Identify three types of enemas and state the purposes of each. _____

   _____

Part 6

Arrange these steps for administering an enema.

1. _____ Apply the clamp and remove the rectal tube when the enema is completed; ask client to retain solution.

2. _____ Place a waterproof pad under the client's buttocks.

3. _____ Separate the client's buttocks and gently insert the rectal tube 3 to 4 inches toward the umbilicus.

4. _____ Assist the client into the bathroom or onto the bedpan with the head of bed elevated.

5. _____ Place the enema bag on an IV pole or raise the container 18 inches above the client's anus.

6. _____ Return the client to a comfortable position.

7. _____ Assist client onto the left side with right knee flexed.

8. _____ Prepare the enema.

9. _____ Hold the tube in place with one hand while opening the clamp with the other hand allowing the solution to flow into the rectum.

10. _____ Close the curtain or door to the room.

52

Specimen Collection

Common Acronyms or Terms

cc	IV
C & S	mL
GI	O & P
I & O	UA

CHAPTER OVERVIEW

Chapter 52 discusses the process of specimen collection and monitoring of intake and output. An overview of techniques for collection of urine, stool, sputum, and blood specimens is provided.

✪ Be sure to review the Learning Objectives from the text.

✔ Be sure to FIRST perform Improving Concentration exercises described in the Introduction before proceeding with the next exercise.

Part 1

Indicate the order in which you find the following major headings in this chapter.

_____ The Sputum Specimen

_____ The Stool Specimen

_____ The Blood Specimen

_____ The Urine Specimen

Part 2

Complete the following statements related to the major headings and key points.

1. Nurses do not draw blood unless they have specific _____ and _____.

2. The major heading The Urine Specimen contains a subheading entitled Testing Urine for _____ Substances.

3. Use body substance _____ when working with body fluids.

4. Routine specimen collection is usually scheduled for _____ in the _____.

Part 3 Key Terms: Knowledge Check

Unscramble the letters to identify the term that best matches the definition.

1. Troxacepete _____
   To spit

2. Doryetherm _____
   Measuring instrument for determining specific gravity; a urinometer

3. Syslainuir _____
   Identification of the components of urine

4. Ciscifep vagytir _____ _____
   Concentration of urine compared with pure water

5. Chomtucel _____
   Method for testing stool for the presence of blood; also known as hematest

6. Unpivecutren _____
   Using a needle to withdraw blood from a vein

Part 4

Answer these statements true (T) or false (F).

1. _____ The amount of fluids a client consumes and eliminates during a given period is an excellent indicator of his or her nutritional and fluid balance.

2. _____ Intake and output refers to fluid intake and does not include solid foods such as Jello.

3. _____ The decimal increments for reading specific gravity are in hundreds.

4. _____ Urine that has a specific gravity of 1.005 is concentrated and is treated with IV fluids.

5. _____ A single-voided urine specimen may be used to test for substances, such as sugar.

6. _____ Before obtaining a sputum specimen, ask the client to brush his or her teeth and use mouthwash.

Part 5

Match the concepts, statements, or definitions in column I with the term, phrase, or number column II. Some answers will not be used.

Column I

1. _____ The client had a 240-mL cup full of ice chips, a styrofoam (120-mL) cup of coffee, and a 4-ounce cup of juice, and voided 250 mL at noon and vomited 120 mL in the emesis basin at 2 PM.

2. _____ A specific gravity of 1.018

3. _____ Process used to obtain a urine specimen from adults, particularly men, to determine the presence of bacteria

4. _____ Used to determine amounts and characteristics of urine during various times of the day

5. _____ A convenient test to measure glucose and acetone at the same time

Column II

a. Clean-catch urine

b. Keto-Diastix

c. Fractional urine specimen

d. 24-hour urine specimen

e. Single-voided specimen

f. Intake: 480 mL; Output: 370 mL

g. Intake: 360 mL; Output: 370 mL

h. Intake: 480 mL; Output: 250 mL

i. Concentrated urine specific gravity

j. Normal specific gravity

Part 6 Short Answer Exercises

Complete the following fill-in-the-blank and short answer questions.

1. To obtain a specimen from a retention catheter, the nurse should _____the drainage tubing and secure it with a rubber band below the _____ port.

2. When beginning the collection of a 24-hour urine specimen, the client should be instructed to void and the nurse should _____ this specimen and record the time on the clent's chart.

3. The best time to collect a sputum specimen is soon after the client _____.

4. When collecting or assisting with the collection of a blood specimen, the nurse should always _____ _____.

5. An accurate stool specimen should include feces from _____ different areas of the stool specimen.

53

Bandages and Binders

Common Acronyms or Terms

ACE

CMS

TED

CHAPTER OVERVIEW

Chapter 53 provides an overview of various bandages and binders. The purpose of using binders and bandages is discussed as well as the techniques for their application.

✪ Be sure to review the Learning Objectives from the text.

✔ Be sure to FIRST perform Improving Concentration exercises described in the Introduction before proceeding with the next exercise.

Part 1

Indicate if the following subheadings are located under the major heading Bandages (Ba) or Binders (Bi).

_____ Antiembolism Stockings

_____ Montgomery Straps

_____ Elastic Roller Bandages

Part 2

Complete the following statements related to the major headings and key points.

1. Never allow an _____

_____ to "bunch up" or cease

circulation in the leg.

2. The subheading Tape is located under the major

heading _____.

3. Binders supply support for specific

_____ _____.

Part 3 Key Terms: Knowledge Check

Match the concepts and definitions in column I with the correct term in column II.

Column I

1. _____ Elastic leg supports used for all postoperative clients; also called TED socks

2. _____ Made of two strips of material, 3 to 4 inches wide, which are fastened together

3. _____ Skin softening and breaking down due to moisture accumulation and lack of circulation

4. _____ A wide, flat piece of fabric that you secure around the trunk of the client's body for support

5. _____ Tape straps used when dressings must be changed often; help prevent skin irritation and maintain skin integrity

Column II

a. Abdominal binder

b. Montgomery straps

c. Antiembolism stockings

d. Maceration

e. T-binder

Part 4 Short Answer Exercises

Complete the short answer questions by filling in the blanks.

1. A bandage is a strip of gauze, cloth, or

_____ material that is wrapped

around a body part to give _____ or to hold _____ in place.

2. Elastic roller bandages are usually wrapped _____ a limb.

3. When applying a binder, apply it _____ enough to give support but not too _____.

4. Before applying large tape dressings, the nurse should _____ the client to reduce painful removal of the tape.

5. Wear _____ when you apply a T-binder. Place the band around the client's _____, and bring the _____ strap _____ the legs, and pin the band and the strip at the _____.

54

Heat and Cold Application

CHAPTER OVERVIEW

Chapter 54 presents an overview of heat and cold application and conditions that might warrant the use of these therapies. Techniques for applying specific heat and cold therapies and rules for application are discussed.

✪ Be sure to review the Learning Objectives from the text.

✔ Be sure to FIRST perform Improving Concentration exercises described in the Introduction before proceeding with the next exercise.

Part 1

Complete the following statements related to the major headings and key points.

1. The subheading under both major headings is

   R _ _ _ _ for A _ _ _ _ _ _ _ _ _ _.

2. The two major headings of the chapter are _ _ _ _

   and _ _ _ _.

3. Heat d _ _ _ _ _ _ surface blood vessels.

4. A s _ _ _ b _ _ _ applies heat and water to the pelvic

   area.

5. Apply moist cold compresses to s _ _ _ _ body parts.

Part 2 Key Terms: Knowledge Check

Match the terms in column I with the definitions in column II.

Column I

1. _____ Ultrasound

2. _____ Hypothermic blanket

3. _____ Infrared rays

4. _____ Ultraviolet rays

5. _____ Icecap

Column II

a. Used to decrease body temperature; used primarily in surgery to prevent complications resulting from unstable temperature regulation

b. A flat, oval, rubber bag with a leakproof screw-in top and wide opening for filling

c. A method of applying deep, penetrating heat to muscles and tissues

d. Mild radiation supplied by sun; used to treat skin infections and wounds

e. These rays relax muscles, stimulate circulation, and relieve pain, and have the same effect as other forms of dry heat.

Part 3

Indicate if the following rules or guidelines for application are for heat (H) or cold (C) therapy.

1. _____ Used to slow or stop bleeding

2. _____ Prolonged exposure to extreme levels may cause frostbite

3. _____ Promotes drainage (draws infected materials out of wounds)

4. _____ Relieves local pain or aching, particularly of muscles or joints

5. _____ Often applied to a sprain, strain, or fracture to help remove blood and lymph congestion

6. _____ Used to control pain and fluid loss in the initial treatment of burns

7. _____ Raises the body's temperature

8. _____ Used to relieve pain in an engorged breast

Part 4 Short Answer and Completions

Complete the following statements by filling in the blanks.

1. Cold application prevents escape of heat from the body by _____ circulation, which also relieves _____ and often relieves muscle pain.

2. When using cold, moist compresses, wring the compress thoroughly and _____ compresses frequently.

3. Fill an icecap about _____ full using small pieces of ice to help the bag fit close to the body.

4. When applying a warm compress to the eye, wash your hands and wear _____ _____ to prevent infecting the eye.

5. Apply _____ _____ to the client's skin before applying a warm moist compress.

6. A warm compress or pack is covered with a dry moisture-proof cover to _____.

7. Cold humidity is often ordered for clients who have _____ difficulties.

8. When giving a tepid sponge bath, place moist cool cloths in the client's _____ and on the _____ because blood vessels lie close to the skin in these areas.

Part 5

Indicate if the following actions are appropriate (A) or inappropriate (I).

1. _____ When giving a tepid sponge bath, use alcohol to quickly bring down a temperature elevation.

2. _____ Give clients who are receiving radiation therapy or chemotherapy warm compresses or hot packs for a longer period of time because these client's need extra warmth for comfort.

3. _____ Before applying an electric heating pad, connect it to an electric outlet and turn the heating switch to high to see whether the pad heats promptly.

4. _____ Inspect the skin of a client receiving heat therapy frequently to prevent burning.

5. _____ Apply a cold pack to an ankle that was sprained 24 hours ago to reduce the swelling that is present.

55

Client Comfort and Pain Management

Common Acronyms or Terms

AHCPR   PCA

JCAHO   TENS

CHAPTER OVERVIEW

Chapter 55 discusses pain management for client comfort. An overview of different types of pain and causes of pain is provided. Techniques for pain management are addressed.

✪ Be sure to review the Learning Objectives from the text.

✔ Be sure to FIRST perform Improving Concentration exercises described in the Introduction before proceeding with the next exercise.

Part 1

Complete the following statements related to the major headings and key points.

1. The major heading in the chapter that has no sub-

    heading is _____ _____.

2. _____ pain lasts more than 6 months.

3. _____ intervention in the

    cycle of pain may help to control it.

4. The major heading Pain Management contains subheadings on pharmacologic and complementary techniques and _____

    _____.

5. Nociception has four components:

    _____, _____,

    _____, and _____

6. To thoroughly assess pain, the nurse should ask the client about what aspects of the pain experience?

    _____

Part 2 Key Terms: Knowledge Check

Review the key terms in the chapter. Match the term in column I and indicate the letter of the correct definition in column II.

Column I

1. _____ Endorphins

2. _____ Guided imagery

3. _____ Intractable

4. _____ Neuropathic pain

5. _____ Analgesics

6. _____ Pain tolerance

7. _____ Nociceptive pain

8. _____ Pain threshold

Column II

a. Discomfort that continues for a long period (6 months or longer), also called chronic pain

b. The lowest intensity of a stimulus that causes a subject to recognize pain

c. Naturally occurring substances produced by the central nervous system that control pain perception

d. The point at which a person can no longer tolerate pain

e. Chronic pain that resists therapeutic intervention

f. Medications that relieve pain

g. Sensation of pain that results abruptly and lasts for 6 months or less; also called acute pain

h. Process through which the client receives a suggestion that helps control the pain

Part 3

Complete the following statements about pain and pain management.

1. The term used to describe normal pain transmission is _____.

2. Activities such as visiting, games, television, or craft projects represent complementary pain control measures called _____ and _____.

3. A great deal of _____ may aggravate pain; a client in pain can benefit by developing effective coping mechanisms.

4. Three classes of analgesics commonly used for pain relief are _____ use for clients with _____ pain, _____ used to manage _____ pain, and _____ used to help improve a client's _____, thus assisting in muscle relaxation.

5. _____ may be needed to alleviate some forms of chronic pain, such as back pain caused by a herniated disk.

Part 4

Indicate if the following actions by a nurse would be appropriate (A) or inappropriate (I).

1. _____ Encourage a client with chronic pain to withdraw from social activities because the stimulation might cause increased discomfort.

2. _____ Explain to clients that acute pain is short term and disappears once the underlying cause is identified and treated.

3. _____ Help a client with chronic pain set goals and target dates to gain control over one part of his or her life at a time to reduce the sense of loss of control that aggravates pain.

4. _____ Encourage the client with chronic pain to join a support group and bond with family when pain is intense.

5. _____ Give pain medication when pain is most intense so that endorphins are present to help the analgesics work more effectively.

6. _____ Tell the client who is 2 weeks postoperative that there should be no pain at this time so what the client is experiencing is probably a memory of previous real pain.

Part 5

Indicate where the following factors fall in the cycle of chronic pain (the first is provided).

1. _____ Muscle tension

2. _____ Fear, stress, conflict lower pain threshold

3. _____ Fatigue makes it difficult to manage pain

4. _____ Lack of knowledge predisposes to more pain

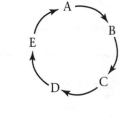

56

Preoperative and Postoperative Care

Common Acronyms or Terms

BP	OR
CBC	PACU
ECG	PAR
I & O	RR
IV	TCDB
NPO	UA
O_2	VS

CHAPTER OVERVIEW

Chapter 56 discusses the client's experience with surgery beginning with preparation and proceeding through the recovery phase. Factors related to surgery including the types of surgery and anesthesia are addressed.

✪ Be sure to review the Learning Objectives from the text.

❧ Be sure to FIRST perform Improving Concentration exercises described in the Introduction before proceeding with the next exercise.

Part 1

Match the subheadings with the major heading under which they can be found.

Column I

1. _____ Assessments
2. _____ Client Transport
3. _____ Anesthesia
4. _____ Postoperative Discomforts
5. _____ Factors in Surgery
6. _____ The Postanesthesia Care Unit

Column II

a. Perioperative Care
b. Preoperative Nursing Care
c. Intraoperative Nursing Care
d. Postoperative Nursing Care

Part 2

Complete the following titles and statements found as major headings and key points.

1. The major heading with no subheadings is _____ Nursing Care.

2. Preoperative _____ is your first line of defense against postoperative complications.

3. Early postoperative complications include hemorrhage, shock, _____, and _____.

4. _____ hygiene is extremely important in the prevention of later postoperative complications.

Part 3 Matching of Key Terms: Knowledge Check

Match the following key terms in the chapter with the appropriate definition.

Column I

1. _____ Embolus
2. _____ Evisceration
3. _____ Dehiscence
4. _____ Splinting

5. _____ Anesthesia

6. _____ Invasive

7. _____ Positive Homans' sign

8. _____ Thrombophlebitis

9. _____ Hypoxia

10. _____ Atelectasis

Column II

a. Process in which an incision is made into the body

b. Pain occurring behind the knee on dorsiflexion; a sign of the presence of thrombophlebitis

c. The complete or partial loss of sensation

d. Decreased blood oxygenation; can result from depressed respiration

e. The collapse of a portion of the lung caused by mucous plugs that close the bronchi

f. Support of the operative area with a pillow to relieve some pain during coughing

g. The opening or separation of the surgical incision

h. Occurs when a piece of a clot breaks off and enters the person's circulatory system, usually ending up in the lungs and causing such complications that death follows

i. The formation of a blood clot in a vein

j. Occurs when the edges of the wound separate and abdominal organs protrude

Part 4

Indicate if the following actions would be appropriate (A) or inappropriate (I) when receiving the postsurgery client in the nursing unit.

1. _____ On receiving a client from the PACU after surgery, keep the client flat, often in Sims' position, until he or she awakens.

2. _____ Clamp all tubes and drains before the PACU nurse leaves your unit.

3. _____ Carry out any orders for immediate drug or oxygen administration.

4. _____ If vomiting occurs, turn the client's head to the side.

5. _____ If the client is receiving IV fluids from the PACU, discontinue infusions and give the client clear liquids to maintain hydration.

Part 5

Circle the letter corresponding to the correct answer.

1. Jane Pathker has returned to you from surgery. You assess her and find she has active reflexes, increased heart rate, irregular breathing, increased BP, pupils widely dilated and divergent. You recognize she is in which stage of general anesthesia?
   a. Stage of analgesia/amnesia
   b. Stage of dreams and excitement
   c. Stage of surgical anesthesia
   d. Stage of toxic or extreme depression

2. Malik Deer, 79 years old, is scheduled for surgery. He has a history of smoking for the past 60 years, weighs 50 pounds over desired weight, and has a large family who will be at the hospital. Which of the following factors make Mr. Deer a high-risk client?
   a. Mr. Deer has factors in the weight, age, and use of chemicals categories.
   b. Mr. Deer has factors in the psychological status category with excessive fear and dementia.
   c. The large family places Mr. Deer at risk because he will likely have excessive stimulation postoperatively.
   d. Being scheduled for surgery puts Mr. Deer at risk because he probably has preexisting physical disorders, a poor hydration status, and electrolyte balance problems from preparations.

3. When teaching Mr. Deer about the preoperative nursing care he will experience, the nurse would explain which of the following?
   a. Directly before the operation, the nurse will see that all specimens and blood samples have been collected and sent to the lab.
   b. On admission to the hospital the day before the operation the nurse will help him to void and document this information on the preoperative checklist form.
   c. Directly before the operation the nurse will remove any complete or partial dentures and place them in a denture cup.
   d. On admission to the hospital until an hour before the operation he will be encouraged to take fluids to prevent dehydration after surgery.

4. Which of the following represents an immediate postoperative complication and the appropriate nursing action to address it?
   a. Nausea which would be treated with sips of cool fluid and an antiemetic such as Compazine
   b. Constipation which would be treated with a stool softener such as docusate (Surfak)
   c. Urinary retention which should be monitored and the client catheterized if not resolved
   d. Hypoxia which is treated by administering oxygen by nasal cannula or mask if necessary

57

Surgical Asepsis

Common Acronyms or Terms

CSR, CSS
OR

CHAPTER OVERVIEW

Chapter 57 discusses sterile technique and surgical asepsis. Differentiation between medical and surgical asepsis is provided. Use of asepsis is demonstrated in an overview of urinary catheterization.

✪ Be sure to review the Learning Objectives from the text.

✔ Be sure to FIRST perform Improving Concentration exercises described in Introduction before proceeding with the next exercise.

Part 1

Indicate the order in which you find the following major headings in this chapter.

1. _____ Sterile Technique
2. _____ Asepsis
3. _____ Urinary Catheterization
4. _____ Disinfection and Sterilization

Part 2

Complete the following statements related to the major headings and key points.

1. _____ applies to medical asepsis. It means the removal of all gross contamination and ____ microorganisms.
2. When a sterile item touches anything unsterile it becomes _____.
3. Client and family teaching is important, especially if the client will need to perform a _____ _____ or catheter care after discharge.
4. The subheadings Hair Covering and Surgical Mask are located under the major heading _____ _____.

Part 3 Key Terms: Knowledge Check

Review the key terms in the chapter. Unscramble the term to reveal the term or terms that best match(es) the definition.

1. Garuscil passise _____ _____
   Destroys all microorganisms
2. Elitrse ecthiquen _____ _____
   Use means that no organisms are carried to the client; used when changing dressing and administering parenteral medications
3. Itryd _____
   Term for an object or person that has not been cleaned or sterilized for removal of microorganisms
4. Coluvatae _____
   Pressure steam sterilizer; allows exposure for 15 minutes to steam under 18 pounds of pressure at a temperature of 257°F (125°C) to kill microorganisms
5. Fistinnocide _____
   Destroys most pathogens but not necessarily their spores

Part 4

Answer these statements true (T) or false (F).

1. _____ A item is sterile if it is free of all microorganisms and spores.

2. _____ The gastrointestinal tract and upper respiratory tract are clean but not sterile.

3. _____ The uterus and urinary bladder are normally clean and easily contaminated.

4. _____ If you are wearing sterile gloves to perform a sterile procedure, keep them close to your body and below the waist to prevent contamination.

5. _____ If you are unsure if you have caused contamination, ask another nurse to check for signs of microorganisms and if none are found you are still sterile.

6. _____ If a sterile wrapper becomes wet, the wrapper and its contents are no longer sterile.

Part 5

Organize the following steps in the skills identified.

A. Putting on Sterile Gloves

_____ Use your nondominant hand to grasp the inside upper surface of the glove's cuff for your dominant hand.

_____ Slip the fingers of your sterile gloved hand under (inside) the cuff of the remaining glove while keeping your thumb pointed outward.

_____ Open the outer glove package on a clean, dry, flat surface at waist level or higher.

_____ Insert your nondominant hand into the glove.

_____ Insert your dominant hand into the glove, placing your thumb and fingers in the proper openings.

B. Catheterizing the Female Client

_____ Put on the clean gloves and wash the woman's perineal area with soap.

_____ Open the sterile catheterization tray on the bedside table.

_____ Close the door or pull the bed curtain.

_____ Ask the client to breath deeply and slowly then insert the catheter gently into her meatus.

_____ With your sterile dominant hand use the forceps to pick up a cotton ball and cleanse both labial folds and then the meatus.

_____ Dry the woman's perineal area if necessary, then remove gloves.

_____ Assist the woman into a supine position with her feet spread apart and her knees flexed.

_____ Pick up the catheter approximately 3 inches from the tip with your sterile dominant hand and place the drainage end in the basin.

_____ Move the catheterization tray with the equipment onto the sterile drape between the client's thighs.

_____ While using your nondominant hand, separate and gently spread the woman's labia minora to expose her urinary meatus.

58

Wound Care

CHAPTER OVERVIEW

Chapter 58 presents an overview of wounds, wound care, and the process of wound healing. Nursing measures to prevent skin breakdown are addressed. Dressing changes and pressure ulcer care are also discussed.

✪ Be sure to review the Learning Objectives from the text.

✔ Be sure to FIRST perform Improving Concentration exercises described in the Introduction before proceeding with the next exercise.

Part 1

Complete the following statements related to the major headings and key points.

1. The two major headings in this chapter are
_____ and _____ .

2. Wounds heal by _____ ,
_____ , or _____
intention.

3. Prevent pressure ulcers by _____
their _____ .

4. A _____ is a disruption in the skin's integrity.

Part 2 Key Terms: Knowledge Check

Match the terms in column I with the definitions in column II.

Column I

1. _____ Sloughing
2. _____ Ischemia
3. _____ Debridement
4. _____ Eschar
5. _____ Laceration
6. _____ Puncture
7. _____ Incision
8. _____ Abrasion
9. _____ Exudate
10. _____ Pressure ulcer

Column II

a. A wound with torn, ragged edges

b. Rubbing off of the skin's surface

c. Removal of infected tissues

d. A stab wound

e. The end results of constant skin pressure; also called bed sores or decubitus

f. Lack of blood supply to tissues

g. Leathery black crust of dead tissue that develops in the fourth stage of wound healing

h. Eschar that separates from living tissue

i. Drainage

j. A wound with clean edges

Part 3

Answer these statements true (T) or false (F).

1. _____ When removing stitches, skin clamps, or staples, clean technique is used because the wound is closed.

2. _____ A wet-to-dry dressing or packing is a common technique for debridement.

3. _____ Moist gauze removes drainage from the ulcer while retaining moisture.

4. _____ Healing by first intention occurs with tissue loss such as deep lacerations or burns.

5. _____ To prevent pressure ulcer formation, massage the client's skin frequently.

6. _____ A pressure ulcer in stage 1 classification has subcutaneous tissue involvement, is not painful, has a foul-smelling drainage, and may require months to heal after pressure is relieved.

Part 4

Indicate if the following activities are appropriate (A) or inappropriate (I).

1. _____ Use clean gloves to remove a soiled dressing from an open wound.

2. _____ Prior to putting on sterile gloves when changing a sterile dressing, open sterile dressings and uncap sterile saline.

3. _____ Position the client to irrigate a wound so that the solution will run from the lower end of the wound toward the upper end.

4. _____ When irrigating a wound, hold the syringe just inside the wound edges to prevent splashing.

5. _____ Teach the client to observe for excess drainage and report severe pain.

Part 5 Short Answer and Completions

Complete the following exercises by filling in the blanks.

1. State the causes and usual locations of pressure ulcers. _____

   _____

2. Indicate an activity the nurse may use to prevent each of the following causes of wound problems:

   Pressure _____

   Shear _____

   Friction _____

   Stripping _____

   Urine or stool _____

   Perspiration _____

   Arterial insufficiency _____

59

Care of the Dying Person

Common Acronyms or Terms

AD

CPR

DNH

DNI

DNR

EEG

IV

PSDA

CHAPTER OVERVIEW

Chapter 59 addresses the dying client and nursing care of the client and family during and after the death. Care of the body after death and coping with a client's death are discussed.

✪ Be sure to review the Learning Objectives from the text.

✔ Be sure to FIRST perform Improving Concentration exercises described in the Introduction before proceeding with the next exercise.

Part 1

Complete the following titles and statements found as major headings and key points.

1. The last two major headings in this chapter are C _ _ _ _ _ for the D_ _ _ P_ _ _ _ _'_ B_ _ _ and C_ _ _ _ _ With a C_ _ _ _ _'_ D_ _ _ _.

2. The heading Care of the Family contains subheadings that include Care as the Person is Dying, Care Following the Death of a Loved One, and The R_ _ _ of H_ _ _ .

3. Changing the dying client's p_ _ _ _ _ _ _ frequently may promote comfort.

4. Pain relief may be necessary to e _ _ _ the dying process.

5. After death, nurses give p_ _ _ _ _ _ _ care to the client's body.

Part 2 Matching of Key Terms: Knowledge Check

Write the term on the line that matches the definition below it.

1. _____
   Fast, labored, and deep breathing; often occurs if a person experiences acidosis

2. _____
   Absence of breathing

3. _____
   Rapid breathing

4. _____
   Postmortem (after death) examination of the body

5. _____
   Alternating periods of absence of breathing and rapid breathing

6. _____
   Formally defined as the irreversible cessation of total brain function, determined by clinical examination; also called brain death

Part 3

Complete these exercises by filling in the blanks.

1. List two nursing interventions that might be performed during the process of dying related to:

   Care of the mouth, nose, and eyes
   _____
   _____
   _____
   _____

   Breathing difficulties _____
   _____
   _____
   _____

   Incontinence _____
   _____
   _____
   _____

   Nutrition _____
   _____
   _____
   _____

   Odor control _____

2. List two signs of approaching death. _____
   _____
   _____
   _____

3. Complete the following statements related to caring for the dead person's body.

   _____ the body and place a
   pillow under the head.

   Remove all _____ bed linens
   but the _____ that covers the
   client.

   _____ all personal belongings,
   and have the family _____ for
   them and take them.

   Send all flowers and cards _____
   with the _____.

Part 4

Match the concepts in column I with the related term or terms in column II.

Column I

1. _____ Expressions of the wishes of clients about the kinds of treatment and care they want to receive at the point of death

2. _____ Do not resuscitate; do not code

3. _____ Do not intubate

4. _____ Designates a person of the client's choice to make healthcare decisions should the client become incompetent in the future

5. _____ A document in which clients state the types of treatment they will accept if a terminal situation arises

Column II

a. Living will

b. Durable power of attorney for healthcare

c. DNI

d. Advance directives

e. DNR

60

Review of Mathematics

Common Acronyms or Terms

cc	mg
G, g, gm	mL
gr	oz
gtt	%
kg	μ
L	

CHAPTER OVERVIEW

Chapter 60 explains the importance of basic mathematics in the administration of medications. Systems of measurement are discussed, as well as methods for converting between different systems. Calculation of drug dosages is addressed.

✪ Be sure to review the Learning Objectives from the text.

✔ Be sure to FIRST perform Improving Concentration exercises described in the Introduction before proceeding with the next exercise.

Part 1 Completions

Complete the sentences by filling in the blanks.

1. According to the major heading Systems of Measurements, the three major systems are _____ Measurement, the _____ System, and the _____ System.

2. The second major heading in the chapter is D_ _ _ _ _ C_ _ _ _ _ _ _ _ _ _ .

3. The nurse must know how to c_ _ _ _ _ _ systems of measurement in the event the d_ _ _ d_ _ _ _ _ is ordered in a different u _ _ _ of m _ _ _ _ _ _ _ _ _ _ than is available for administration.

4. Four major subheadings under Dosage Calculation include R_ _ _ _s and P_ _ _ _ _ _ _ _s, F_ _ _ _ _ _ _s, S_ _ _ _ _ _ _ _ _ F_ _ _ _s, and P_ _ _ _ _ _ _ _ _.

Part 2

Match the unit of measurement in column I with the system of measurement in column II.

Column I

1. _____ Teaspoon
2. _____ Milligram
3. _____ Minim
4. _____ Drop
5. _____ Pint
6. _____ Liter

Column II

a. Metric
b. Household
c. Apothecaries'

Part 3

Match the prefix in column I with the appropriate meaning listed in column II.

Column I

1. _____ Deci

2. _____ Kilo

3. _____ Deca

4. _____ Micro

5. _____ Centi

Column II

a. Multiply by 10; ×10

b. Multiply by 100; ×100

c. Divide by 100; 1/100

d. Divide by 1,000; 1/1,000

e. Divide by 10; 1/10

f. Divide by 1,000,000; 1/millionth

Part 4 Short Answer Exercises

Complete the following short answer questions.

1. If you need grams of a medication and you have the medication in milligrams, how would you convert the amount? _____

2. List the steps involved in dividing fractions._____

3. In a fraction, the larger denominator denotes _____ pieces. Therefore, 1/100 is _____ as much as 1/50.

4. What can nurses do if unsure about their dosage calculations? _____

Part 5 Multiple Choice

Circle the letter corresponding to the correct answer.

1. The doctor ordered aspirin 1/100 gr. You have tablets of aspirin that are 1/200 gr each. You would administer _____ tablet(s).
   a. One-half
   b. One
   c. Two
   d. Five

2. The doctor orders 3,000 mL of IV fluid for Mr. Peters. The first hour Mr. Peters is to receive 30% of the fluid. How much should you administer over the first hour?
   a. 30 mL
   b. 90 mL
   c. 300 mL
   d. 900 mL

3. The doctor orders 60 mg Tylenol. You have on hand Tylenol elixir 120 mg/5 mL. How much would you administer?
   a. 0.25 mL
   b. 2.5 mL
   c. 5 mL
   d. 50 mL

4. You must administer 2 teaspoons of syrup of Ipecac. You have available a 20-mL syringe and the syrup. How much would you administer in the syringe?
   a. 0.1 mL
   b. 1.0 mL
   c. 10 mL
   d. 20 mL

5. You must infuse a 250-mL bag of gentamicin at a rate of 50 mL/hr. How long will it take you to administer the full amount?
   a. 5 hours
   b. 2.5 hours
   c. 0.5 hours
   d. 0.25 hours

61

Introduction to Pharmacology

Common Acronyms or Terms

CNM	NP
DDS	OTC
DEA	PDR
DO	RPh
DVM	TO
FDA	USD
MD	USP
NF	VO
NIH	WWW

CHAPTER OVERVIEW

Chapter 61 discusses pharmacology and the nursing considerations related to the properties of medications. Legal concerns related to medication storage and administration are discussed. An overview of dosage orders and prescriptions is provided.

✪ Be sure to review the Learning Objectives from the text.

✔ Be sure to FIRST perform Improving Concentration exercises described in the Introduction before proceeding with the next exercise.

Part 1

Indicate the order in which you find the following major headings in this chapter.

_____ How Medications Are Prescribed

_____ Legal Aspects

_____ Medication Preparations and Actions

Part 2

Complete the following statements related to the major headings and key points.

1. A nurse may obtain information concerning medications from _____ _____ and computer _____, which are common sources of information.

2. The three subheadings found in this chapter under Medication Preparations and Actions are Medication: _____, _____, and _____.

Part 3 Key Terms: Knowledge Check

Review the key terms in the chapter. Mark (y) beside the terms you recognize and can define and (n) beside the terms you do not know. List the terms marked with an (n) in the spaces below and write an abbreviated definition of each term as you read.

Term

_____

_____

_____

_____

_____

Definition

_____

_____

_____

_____

_____

Part 4

Unscramble the letters to identify the term or terms that best match(es) the definition.

1. Eedasog _____
   A single amount of a medication and scheduled time

2. Drastelmarn _____
   Medications given in this form are absorbed through the skin

3. Holmacpyrogm _____
   Science that deals with the origin, nature, chemistry, effects, and uses of medications

4. Trecine-datoce _____
   Cover of medication does not dissolve until tablet reaches the intestine

5. Pletac _____
   Tablet in the shape of a capsule

Part 5

Answer these questions true (T) or false (F).

1. _____ The nurse should not reveal possible side effects of a medication to a client to avoid causing the client to thinking those symptoms into reality.

2. _____ The Federal Food, Drug, and Cosmetic Act ensures that medications and therapeutic agents are safe and effective for public use.

3. _____ A scheduled drug count verification means each nurse going off duty should count all the routine medications for their client and verify that the next shift's dosages are ready to administer.

4. _____ Controlled substances that are schedule II, III, or IV are locked up; all use is documented.

5. _____ The *Physician's Desk Reference (PDR)* is kept on most nursing units as a reference.

Part 6

Match the concepts and definitions in column I with the terms in column II.

Column I

1. _____ Medication that produces a desired response

2. _____ Form of medication that can be administered orally, parenterally, or topically

3. _____ A medication in powdered form enclosed in soluble, cylindrical, gelatin-like material

4. _____ 2-(4-isobutylphenyl) propionic acid is the _____ for ibuprofen.

5. _____ A medication that has an opposing effect or acts against another medication

6. _____ A compressed, spherical form of a medication

7. _____ Motrin, Nuprin, or Advil are _____ for ibuprofen.

8. _____ A synergistic effect; enhances the effects of another medication

9. _____ The amount of medication required to obtain a desired effect in the majority of clients

10. _____ A written formula for preparing and giving a medication

Column II

a. Capsule

b. Prescription

c. Therapeutic dose

d. Tablet

e. Agonist

f. Trade/brand name

g. Potentiating effect

h. Antagonist

i. Chemical name

j. Liquid

Part 7 Short Answer Exercises

Complete these short answer questions by filling in the blanks.

1. List three things the nurse should know about the medication being administered. _____

   _____

   _____

   _____

2. Parenteral administration routes include _____, _____, _____, or _____ injections.

3. List four factors healthcare professionals must consider when prescribing medication.

   _____

   _____

   _____

   _____

62

Classification of Medications

Common Acronyms or Terms

ACE	NSAID
ANS	OTC
ASA	PCN
b.i.d.	PPF
CA	PRN
C & S	PT
CNS	PTT
DM	q.d.
GI	q.i.d.
HCl	SO_4
HS	SSKI
MOM	t.i.d.
MS	

CHAPTER OVERVIEW

Chapter 62 discusses the system by which medications are classified and implications for the nurse in medication administration. Major drug classifications are discussed with an overview of primary drug types within these classifications.

✪ Be sure to review the Learning Objectives from the text.

✔ Be sure to FIRST perform Improving Concentration exercises described in the Introduction before proceeding with the next exercise.

Part 1

Unscramble the following words to reveal some of the major headings in this chapter.

1. *Nopaslicinteat* Medications _____

2. Medications That Affect the *Tuimengaytern* System

_____ _____

3. *Tiboniactis* and Other *Nait-ficenivet* Agents

_____

Part 2

Complete the following statements related to the major headings and key points.

1. When seeking information concerning medications, the nurse should use the most

c_____ d_____

r_____ available.

2. The fourth major heading is Medications That Affect the E_____ System.

Part 3

Fill in the term or terms that best match(es) the definition.

1. _____
   Antibiotic agents that kill bacteria

2. _____
   Neurotransmitters that play an important part in the body's response to stress

3. _____
   Medication that has a calming or quieting effect

4. _____
   Medication that produces sleep; usually taken at bedtime

5. _____
   Medications used to relieve constipation; a laxative agent

Part 4

Match the commonly prescribed medication in column I with the classification listed in column II.

Column I

1. _____ tetracycline
2. _____ lanolin
3. _____ diazepam (Valium)
4. _____ morphine (Morphine Sulfate)
5. _____ dexamethasone (Decadron)
6. _____ captopril (Capoten)
7. _____ lidocaine (Xylocaine)
8. _____ aminophylline (Aminophyllin)
9. _____ pseudoephedrine (Sudafed)
10. _____ dimenhydrinate (Dramamine)

Column II

a. Antiarrhythmic

b. Antiemetic

c. Antibiotic anti-infective

d. Bronchodilator

e. Adrenal gland medication

f. Decongestant

g. Sedative/hypnotic

h. Dermatologic

i. Narcotic

j. Antihypertensive

Part 5

Identify the action, use, and two major side effects for the classification/medication below.

Classification/ Medication	Action/Use	Side Effects
1. Penicillins (amox-icillin/Amoxil)	_____	_____
2. Hypnotics (pheno-barbital/Luminal)	_____	_____
3. NSAIDs (nonster-oidal anti-inflam-matory drugs)	_____	_____
4. Adrenergic medica-		

tions (epinephrine/ _____ _____
Adrenaline)

5. Steroids (predni- _____ _____
sone/Delta-Cortef)

Part 6 Short Answer Exercise

Complete these statements by filling in the blanks.

1. If an antibiotic is used indiscriminately, or is administered improperly, organisms may become a_____-r_____.

2. S_____ speed up certain mental and physical processes; d_____ slow them down.

3. State five cushingoid side effects that might occur with prolonged steroid use. _____
_____

Part 7 Multiple Choice Exercises

Circle the letter corresponding to the correct answer.

1. You have a client who has infected rat bites. The doctor orders medications to treat the infection. As you check the medications sent up by pharmacy you would question which of the following as a possible error?
   a. cefazolin (Kefzol)
   b. amoxicillin (Trimox)
   c. theophylline
   d. cotrimoxazole/trimethoprim and sulfamethoxa-zole (Septra, Bactrim)

2. Gil Jones is admitted from home. He has been taking digitalis (Digoxin) for the past 6 months. He has complaints of nausea, blurred vision, and constipation. The monitor shows atrial fibrillation. You recognize that:
   a. Atrial fibrillation is a sign of digitalis toxicity
   b. Blurred vision is a sign Mr. Jones needs additional digitalis
   c. Constipation is a sign Mr. Jones needs a digitalizing dose
   d. The nausea is a sign of digitalis toxicity

3. You administer 20 mg morphine to your client Sean Penn following a cast application for a broken arm. You later notice he is drowsy, his pulse is 65/min, respirations 6/min, and his pupils are constricted. You realize that:

a. Respiratory rate indicates a dangerous side effect of morphine
b. Pulse rate indicates he needs a higher dose of morphine
c. Constriction of the pupils is an unexpected effect of the morphine
d. Drowsiness is a sign that the morphine is having a negative effect

4. The common side effects of thyroid replacement hormones include:
   a. Somnolence
   b. Palpitations
   c. Bradycardia
   d. Urinary retention

63

Administration of Medications

Common Acronyms or Terms

D$_5$W	NG
D$_5$W/2NS	NS
D$_5$NS	OD
DRF	OS
GT	OU
gtt	PICC
HS	PO
ID	PRN
IM	R, PR
IV	SL
IVPB	STAT
JT	subQ
MAR	TD
mg	TPN
mL	V
NaCl	

CHAPTER OVERVIEW

Chapter 63 discusses the storage, preparation, and administration of medications. Safety concerns in medication administration are also discussed. Medication administration by different routes is addressed.

☼ Be sure to review the Learning Objectives from the text.

✔ Be sure to FIRST perform Improving Concentration exercises described in the Introduction before proceeding with the next exercise.

Part 1

Match the subheadings with the following major headings under which they are found.

Column I

1. _____ Medication Errors

2. _____ Local and Systemic Effects

3. _____ Administration by Injection

4. _____ Setting Up Medications

5. _____ Noninjection Methods

6. _____ Sublingual Administration

Column II

a. Preparation

b. Safety

c. General Principles of Medication Administration

d. Enteral Administration Methods

e. Parenteral Administration Methods

Part 2

Unscramble the letters to identify the term or terms that best match(es) the definition.

1. Vasdere effect _____ effect
   Side effect; a response that is not intended or desired

2. Tarnilifiton _____
   Intravenous solution infuses into tissues instead of the vein

3. Farnistonus _____
   Administration of blood or blood products intravenously

4. Paclynacathi _____
   Severe life-threatening allergic reaction to a medication

5. Ixcotyti _____
   Undesired, harmful effect that results from an increased blood level of the medication beyond its therapeutic level

Part 3

Complete the following by filling in the blanks.

1. A nurse documents administration of medications

   on a _____ _____

   (MAR), often a computer-generated sheet prepared

   by the pharmacy.

2. A medication's effects may be _____

   or _____.

3. State the five rights of medication administration.

   _____

   _____

4. _____ administration is ad-

   ministration of medications into any part of the

   body other than the gastrointestinal tract.

Part 4

Answer these questions true (T) or false (F).

1. _____ A STAT order means that the medication
   should be given subcutaneously twice at a
   time.

2. _____ A PRN medication should be given per regular interval.

3. _____ If a client refuses a medication the nurse
   should explain the importance of the medication to the client, then document that
   the medication was refused and dispose of it.

4. _____ When drawing up medication you should
   hold an ampule upright, and tap on the ampule's stem or hold the ampule by the stem
   and rotate your hand in a circular motion.

5. _____ If a client has diseased muscle with poor tissue perfusion, IM injections should be given
   to that area so that the medication will have
   a local and systemic effect on the muscle.

Part 5

Replace the abbreviations in the sentences below with the correct terms.

1. The doctor ordered *TPN* to be given by *IV* through

   the client's *PICC* line. _____

2. If the client complains of chest pain, the nurse

   should administer the cardiac drug *STAT* either *TD*

   by patch or *S* by pill. _____

3. The nurse began to prepare the *IVPB* antibiotic but

   stopped for a moment to find the *DRF* for the tub-

   ing. _____ _____

Part 6

*Match the definitions in column I with the route in col-
umn II and the administration method in column III (answer should contain two letters; column III letters may be
used more than once).*

Column I

1. _____ Medications are placed under the tongue
   where they are dissolved and absorbed.

2. _____ Medications are shallow and given just beneath the epidermis.

3. _____ Medication is administered into adipose tissues located below the dermis.

4. _____ Medication is placed between the client's
   cheek and gum.

5. _____ Medication is introduced directly into the
   bloodstream; medication is absorbed rapidly.

Column II

a. Buccal

b. Sublingual

c. Intravenous

d. Intradermal

e. Subcutaneous

Column III

f. Enteral

g. Parenteral

Part 7

Order the steps of the following skills correctly.

1. Nursing Procedure 63-1 Administering Oral Medications

_____ Prepare all medications, then compare each one again to the medication order.

_____ Record medication administration on the appropriate form.

_____ Check the client's name on the identification bracelet.

_____ Gather equipment and use the MAR to verify the medication order.

_____ Remain with the client until he or she has taken all medication.

_____ Select the correct medication from the drawer or shelf.

2. Nursing Procedure 63-2 Drawing Up a Medication From a Vial

_____ Use your dominant hand to pull back on the syringe's plunger. Withdraw an accurate dose into the syringe.

_____ Hold the needle and recheck the syringe's content for presence of air. Tap the barrel of the syringe to move air bubbles upward prior to expelling them.

_____ Invert the vial, brace your little finger against the plunger.

_____ Insert the needle through the center of the rubber stopper and inject air into the vial, keeping the needle above the solution.

_____ Remove the needle cap and add the amount of air to the syringe equal to the amount of medication that you will withdraw from the vial; change the needle if necessary, recap the needle or pull the safety sheath over it.

3. Nursing Procedure 63-3 Giving a Subcutaneous Injection

_____ Hold the syringe in your dominant hand like a pencil or dart.

_____ Release the skin and move your nondominant hand to steady the syringe's lower end.

_____ Aspirate for a blood return by pulling back on the plunger with your dominant hand.

_____ Record the medication administration indicating that you used the subcutaneous site.

_____ Remove the needle cap; use your nondominant hand to gently bunch or spread tissue at the injection site.

_____ Massage the site gently with the alcohol swab unless contraindicated for the specific medication.

_____ Assist the client to a comfortable position. Select the appropriate site using anatomic landmarks.

_____ Insert the needle quickly at the correct angle (45° for ⅝-inch needle).

_____ Inject the medication at a slow and steady rate.

_____ Put on gloves and close the door or pull the bed curtains.

64

Normal Pregnancy

Common Acronyms or Terms

BPM	FAS	OB
DES	FHT	RhoGAM
EDC	G, P	TPAL
EDD	HG	

CHAPTER OVERVIEW

Chapter 64 discusses the process of pregnancy beginning with issues before and including conception. An overview of preparations for parenthood is provided.

✪ Be sure to review the Learning Objectives from the text.

✔ Be sure to FIRST perform Improving Concentration exercises described in the Introduction before proceeding with the next exercise.

Part 1

Indicate whether the following headings are major (Ma) or minor (Mi).

_____ Fetal Development

_____ Pregnancy and Gestation

_____ Teratogenic Factors

_____ Natural Childbirth

_____ Antepartal Care

_____ Preparing for Parenthood

Part 2

Complete the following statements by filling in the blanks.

1. A _____ is an environmental agent or factor that causes defects in the fetus.

2. _____ refers to the period between conception and the onset of labor.

3. In general, the pregnant woman should _____ daily routines that promote good health.

Part 3 Key Terms: Knowledge Check

Match the statement in column I with the closely related term or concept in column II.

Column I

1. _____ A morula or decidua once it is fully implanted

2. _____ A definite pigmentation of the abdomen often appears as a dark line extending from the umbilicus to the pubis.

3. _____ The developing organism after the eighth week in the 40-week system

4. _____ A fluid-filled sac in which the fetus floats

5. _____ A vascular and glandular organ that supplies the developing organism with food and oxygen, carries waste away to the woman, and produces hormones that help maintain pregnancy

6. _____ A hollow ball of developing cells with an inner and outer layer of cells

7. _____ Means that the fetus is mature enough to survive outside the uterus; usually 24 weeks

8. _____ Excess of amniotic fluid

9. _____ Total time from the moment of fertilization of the egg until birth of the newborn

10. _____ A suntanned, bronzed masking across the face of dark-haired pregnant women

Column II

a. Embryo

b. Fetus

c. Placenta

d. Amnion

e. Viability

f. Chorion

g. Gestation

h. Chloasma

i. Linea nigra

j. Hydramnios

Part 4

Answer these statements true (T) or false (F).

1. _____ Life begins when the ovum is fertilized by the sperm.

2. _____ Amenorrhea and nausea are positive signs of pregnancy.

3. _____ Quickening is a presumptive sign of pregnancy.

4. _____ Hegar's sign and ballottement are probable signs of pregnancy.

5. _____ Fetal heart tones heard distinctly are a presumptive sign of pregnancy.

Part 5

Fill in the term or terms that best match(es) the definition.

1. _____
First fetal movements that the expectant woman feels

2. _____
Nausea or vomiting occurring in pregnancy that lasts beyond the fourth month

3. _____
Abnormal craving for nonfood items during pregnancy

4. _____
Rebound reaction that occurs with gentle tapping of the pregnant woman's abdomen

Part 6

Complete the following statements by filling in the blanks.

1. The pregnant woman needs an increase in caloric intake by approximately _____ calories

2. If a woman experiences constipation, she may take a stool _____ or increase _____ to prevent constipation; however, _____ and enemas should be avoided.

3. A woman should bathe as usual and use minimal or little _____ on her nipples.

4. Sexual intercourse during pregnancy is _____ _____ as long as it is not unduly uncomfortable.

5. Most teratogenic effects occur in the _____ trimester of pregnancy.

6. _____ _____ is the most common discomfort of early pregnancy that may be relieved with _____ _____ meals and _____ carbohydrate foods.

7. Ideal family-centered care begins with _____ for _____.

8. _____ _____ are held for the expectant father and mother together.

9. _____ _____ is a broad term used for management of labor.

10. A woman's feelings about her pregnancy are likely to be influenced by her personal _____ and the _____ and _____ support she receives from family and others close to her.

65

Normal Labor, Delivery, and Postpartum Care

Common Acronyms or Terms

AROM

BPM

FHT

RhoGAM

SROM

SVE

CHAPTER OVERVIEW

Chapter 65 discusses the delivery and postpartum aspects of the birth process beginning with the stages of labor. Nursing care during the stages of labor and postpartum is addressed.

✪ Be sure to review the Learning Objectives from the text.

✔ Be sure to FIRST perform Improving Concentration exercises described in the Introduction before proceeding with the next exercise.

Part 1

Unscramble the following words to reveal some of the major headings in this chapter.

1. *Roalb* _____

2. *Denosc* Stage _____

3. *Topputrasm* Care _____

Part 2

Complete the following statements related to the key points.

1. The onset of true labor may be difficult to _____, even for the multigravida.

2. The third stage is the _____ of the _____.

3. In the postpartum woman, major _____ occur in most body systems, restoring them to their normal prepregnant state.

4. Breasts will begin producing milk within __ to __ days postpartum.

Part 3

Fill in term or terms that best match(es) the definitions.

1. _____
   The settling of the fetus lower into the pelvis; "baby has dropped"

2. _____
   Thin yellowish secretion that provides vitamins and immune bodies

3. _____
   The cervical os begins to open; measured in centimeters

4. _____
   Thinning of the cervix

5. _____
   Painful cramps that occur for a few days after delivery as the uterine muscles contract

6. _____
   Top of the fetal head appears

Part 4

Match the occurrence described in column I with the related stage listed in column II. Letters may be used more than once.

Column I

1. _____ The placenta is delivered.

2. _____ Cervix dilates to 6 cm.

3. _____ Crowning occurs; the nurse instructs the woman to pant.

4. _____ Show is noted, fetal monitoring is done externally or internally.

5. _____ Lochia flow is bright red, and moderate; nurse checks perineal pads.

6. _____ The baby is delivered; the nurse wraps the child and takes it to the parents.

7. _____ The placenta moves into the vagina; the nurse massages the fundus of the uterus.

8. _____ The woman complains of feeling chilled and shakes uncontrollably; the nurse provides blankets and encourages bonding with the child.

Column II

a. First stage of labor

b. Second stage of labor

c. Third stage of labor

d. Fourth stage of labor

Part 5

Complete these sentences by filling in the blanks.

1. If the membranous sac breaks without medical intervention, it is termed _____ _____ of _____ (SROM); if the birth attendant breaks the membrane it is termed _____ _____ of _____ (AROM).

2. The normal lie of the fetus is _____; in a _____ lie the fetus is lying crosswise in the uterus and cannot be delivered in that position.

3. The first stage of labor has a _____ phase in which the contractions occur every 5 to 20 minutes and last 30 to 50 seconds; an _____ phase in which contractions occur every 2 to 4 minutes and last 45 to 60 seconds; and a _____ phase in which contractions occur every 2 to 3 minutes and last 60 to 90 seconds.

4. List five danger signs in labor. _____

_____

_____

_____

5. The midwife notes that the fetal head is at the level of the ischial spines. This means the head is at _____ station and is said to be _____.

6. List three differences between true labor and false labor.

_____

_____

_____

_____

_____

66

Care of the Normal Newborn

Common Acronyms or Terms

G6PD

PKU

SIDS

CHAPTER OVERVIEW

Chapter 66 presents an overview of the characteristics of and nursing care for the normal newborn. Newborn assessment and client teaching are addressed.

✪ Be sure to review the Learning Objectives from the text.

✔ Be sure to FIRST perform Improving Concentration exercises described in the Introduction before proceeding with the next exercise.

Part 1

Complete the following statements related to the major headings and key points.

1. Many reflex behaviors are necessary for the newborn to _____ once outside the uterus.

2. The second major heading of the chapter discusses the _____ of the Newborn.

3. Complete the title of the major heading in the chapter that has no subheading: D _ _ _ _ _ _ _.

4. Accurate newborn assessment requires information from _____ through _____ periods.

5. _____ _____ is the most appropriate food for infants because it provides protection from some infections and diseases.

Part 2 Key terms: Knowledge Check

Fill in the line with the term(s) defined below them.

1. _____
   A white, thick, cheesy material that may cover the skin of a newborn

2. _____
   Accumulation of fluid within the newborn's scalp, caused by pressure to the head during delivery

3. _____
   Fine downy hair seen on the face, shoulders, and back of a newborn

Part 3 Key Terms: Knowledge Check

Match the terms in column I with the definitions in column II.

Column I

1. _____ Pseudomenstruation

2. _____ Acrocyanosis

3. _____ Fontanels

4. _____ Cephalhematoma

5. _____ Desquamate

6. _____ Phimosis

7. _____ Phenylketonuria

8. _____ Galactosemia

Column II

a. Peel

b. Inherited disorder caused by the body's inability to digest protein normally

c. Hereditary disease in which the newborn cannot digest galactose

d. Small amount of bloody mucus expelled from the vagina of the female newborn

e. The foreskin covers the glans penis or extends beyond it with an opening that is very small.

f. Newborn extremities appear cyanotic because of slow peripheral circulation.

g. Accumulation of blood between the bones of the skull and the periosteum

h. Soft spots in the newborn's skull

Part 4

Answer these statements true (T) or false (F).

1. _____ Bonding is the promotion of attachment between parents and newborns.

2. _____ Pinhead-sized white spots on the nose and cheeks of a newborn indicate facial infection.

3. _____ The newborn's cord stump should be kept moist with sterile water to help it to heal.

4. _____ The Babinski reflex should be absent in the newborn; fanning of the big toe is abnormal.

5. _____ Sudden noise or jarring should cause the newborn to throw out the arms and draw up legs.

Part 5 Short Answer and Completions

Complete the following exercises by filling in the blanks.

1. The immediate assessment of the newborn involves: _____, newborn's _____ and _____, and complete _____ _____ on admission to newborn nursery.

2. The Apgar score is obtained at _____ minute and _____ minutes after birth

3. A child with a heart rate of 90, slow irregular respiratory effort, active motion, vigorous cry, and completely pink color would have an Apgar score of _____ and would need _____ resuscitation.

4. A newborn who has respiratory distress might reveal what signs (name three)? _____ _____ _____ _____ _____

5. The nurse who delays the first bath until the newborn's temperature is 98.6°F, then bathes the newborn under a radiant heater and initially leaves the vernix on is trying to prevent _____ _____.

6. When does the newborn receive an identification band? _____ _____ _____ _____

67

High-Risk Pregnancy and Childbirth

Common Acronyms or Terms

AFP	HG	PIH
CD	IV	PROM
CPD	LOP	PUBS
CVS	LS	RhoGAM
D & C	MgSO$_4$	ROP
FBP	MSAFP	STD
FHT	NPO	SVE
GDM	NST	US
HELLP	OCT	
Hg	OP	

CHAPTER OVERVIEW

Chapter 67 discusses complications that may occur with pregnancy from conception through delivery. Maternal disorders as well as fetal concerns, including death, are addressed. The nurse's role with high-risk pregnancy and childbirth is discussed.

✪ Be sure to review the Learning Objectives from the text.

✔ Be sure to FIRST perform Improving Concentration exercises described in the Introduction before proceeding with the next exercise.

Part 1

In what order would you find the following major headings in the chapter?

_____ Complications of Labor and Delivery

_____ When the Newborn Dies

_____ Interrupted Pregnancy

_____ Complications During Pregnancy

_____ Complications of the Postpartum Period

Part 2 Key Terms: Knowledge Check

Review the key terms in the chapter. Most of following definitions or statements are incorrect. Correct the word(s), when needed, to make all definitions/statements accurate.

1. *Dystocia* means outside; a dystocic pregnancy implants outside the uterus.
2. *Hydramnios* refers to a condition in which hypertension, edema, and proteinuria occur during pregnancy.
3. *Gestational diabetes* is one of the most severe complications of pregnancy; involves tonic-clonic seizures.
4. *Preeclampsia* occurs when a woman develops either edema, proteinuria, or both, usually after the 20th week of gestation.
5. *Polyhydramnios* is excessive amniotic fluid and presents serious dangers to the fetus.

Part 3

Indicate if the following actions are appropriate (A) or inappropriate (I).

1. _____ Inserting a sterile gloved hand into the vagina to hold the fetal presenting part away from a prolapsed cord

2. _____ Administering anti-D gamma globulin (RhoGAM) to the Rh-negative woman

3. _____ Instructing the woman with preeclampsia to lie on her right side as much as possible

4. _____ Monitoring a woman for whom a multiple pregnancy is expected for precipitate delivery

5. _____ Recognizing that a woman with blood pressure of 180/120, weight gain of 7 pounds over the past 7 days, and a urine output of 20 mL/hr has preeclampsia and should go home and rest

Part 4

Fill in the term or terms that best match(es) the definition.

1. _____
   Nonabsorbable suture; holds the cervix closed during the remainder of the pregnancy

2. _____
   Insertion of a needle through the maternal abdominal wall into the amniotic sac and withdrawal of amniotic fluid

3. _____
   Condition when the placenta implants in the lower segment of the uterus, rather than in the upper wall

4. _____
   Sudden premature separation of the normally implanted placenta from the uterine wall

5. _____
   Prolonged, painful labor that does not result in effective cervical dilation or effacement

Part 5

Match the concepts in column I with the term or terms in column II.

Column I

1. _____ The embryo dies in utero, and the chorionic villi degenerate, forming grape-like clusters of vesicles.

2. _____ Manual rotation of the fetus before engagement

3. _____ Can arise if the woman's blood type is O and the fetus's is a A, B, or AB

4. _____ A way to evaluate the response of the fetal heart to contractions

5. _____ The umbilical cord wrapped around the fetus's neck

Column II

a. Nuchal cord

b. ABO incompatibility

c. Oxytocic challenge test (OCT)

d. Hydatidiform mole

e. Version

68

The High-Risk Newborn

Common Acronyms or Terms

AGA	LGA
AIDS	NEC
CMV	NICU
DS	PKU
EF	PO_2
FAS	PT
H_2O	RDS
HIV	SGA
HSV	SIDS
LBW	VLBW

CHAPTER OVERVIEW

Chapter 68 discusses the newborn with a complication. Characteristics of the compromised or high-risk infant are presented. The nurse's role in care of the vulnerable newborn, the mother, and the family is addressed.

✪ Be sure to review the Learning Objectives from the text.

✔ Be sure to FIRST perform Improving Concentration exercises described in the Introduction before proceeding with the next exercise.

Part 1

Complete the following statements related to the major headings and key points.

1. The third and fourth major headings in the chapter are: _____ _____, and _____ _____.

2. The subheadings Cocaine and Crack and Heroin are found under the major heading: The _____ _____ _____.

3. Nurses are commonly the first to observe signs of drug _____ in newborns.

4. The newborn may acquire an infection while in the uterus, during _____, during _____, or while in the _____.

5. Identifying risk situations affecting the woman and newborn is vitally important to adequate ____ _____.

Part 2 Key Terms: Knowledge Check

Review the key terms in the chapter. Unscramble the term in column I and indicate the letter of the correct definition in column II.

Column I

1. Hecpanlynea _____

2. Sapisidape _____

3. Hurtsh _____

4. Asinp ibadif _____

5. Dephryshulaco _____

Column II

a. A congenital anomaly in which the vertebral spaces fail to close, allowing a herniation of the spinal contents into a sac

b. Caused by an overabundance of cerebrospinal fluid in the brain's ventricles

c. When the urethral meatus is located on the upper side of the penis

d. Newborn in whom all or part of the brain is missing

e. Yeast infection, in which milklike spots form in the newborn's mouth

Part 3

Answer these statements true (T) or false (F).

1. _____ Erythroblastosis fetalis is a hemolytic condition that occurs when an Rh-negative mother gives birth to an Rh-positive baby.

2. _____ Intracranial hemorrhage is a congenital disorder in which the child has trisomy 21 and demonstrates slanted eyes, large tongue, and several other cardinal signs.

3. _____ Exstrophy of the bladder is a congenital disorder in which there is an abnormal development of the bladder, abdominal wall, and symphysis pubis.

4. _____ Human immunodeficiency virus (HIV) is acquired by infants primarily through sexual abuse from an infected person.

5. _____ Toxoplasmosis is found in cat feces and in rare or raw meat.

Part 4

Indicate if the following actions by a nurse would be appropriate (A) or inappropriate (I).

1. _____ Keeping environmental stimuli to a minimum when caring for a chemically dependent newborn

2. _____ Monitoring for symptoms including lethargy, poor feeding, and jitteriness as signs that a newborn is experiencing withdrawal from cocaine or crack

3. _____ Recognizing that microcephaly, being small for gestational age, and mental retardation are possible effects of cytomegalovirus on the newborn

4. _____ Informing a mother that her baby, whose birth weight is below the 10th percentile expected for that gestational age, is appropriate for gestational age (AGA) but very low birth weight.

5. _____ Bathing a preterm newborn immediately after birth to remove skin organisms and prevent infection

6. _____ Providing the premature newborn with 2-hour feedings until the newborn tolerates 15 mL at each feeding

Part 5

Complete the following by filling in the blanks.

1. _____-for-gestational age newborns are born most often to mothers with diabetes, and usually experience _____ when born as the newborn quickly uses all available carbohydrates.

2. List three potential complications in the high-risk newborn. _____

_____

_____

3. Discuss the nursing actions needed for the premature newborn related to possible ineffective breathing pattern. _____

_____

_____

4. List two chemicals a newborn may be born dependent on and the effects of the use of the drug during pregnancy on the newborn. _____

_____

_____

69

Sexuality, Fertility, and Sexually Transmitted Diseases

Common Acronyms or Terms

AIDS	IVF
CMV	Pap
FTA-ABS	PID
HIV	RPR
HPV	STD
HSV	VDRL
IUD	

CHAPTER OVERVIEW

Chapter 69 discusses human sexuality including sexual orientation, fertility issues, and sexually transmitted diseases. The role of the nurse in addressing issues related to sexuality and fertility is also discussed.

✪ Be sure to review the Learning Objectives from the text.

✔ Be sure to FIRST perform Improving Concentration exercises described in the Introduction before proceeding with the next exercise.

Part 1

Indicate the order in which you find the following major headings in this chapter.

_____ Fertility Control

_____ Human Sexuality

_____ Sexually Transmitted Diseases

_____ Infertility

Part 2

Complete the following statements related to the major headings and key points.

1. Human sexuality involves the whole body, _____, and _____. It is at the _____ of each individual's personality.

2. The two subheadings found in this chapter under Infertility, other than Male and Female Infertility, are _____ _____ and _____.

3. Sexual dysfunction is a person's inability to _____ or _____ in sexual activity for any reason.

Part 3 Key Terms: Knowledge Check

Identify the term or terms that best match(es) the definition.

1. _____
   Method of birth control

2. _____
   Inability to achieve or sustain an erection

3. _____
   Culmination of sexual excitement

4. _____
   Continued erection accompanied by pain

5. _____
   Painful intercourse

Part 4

Match the descriptions/definitions in column I with the terms in column II.

Column I

1. _____ Individuals who are attracted to the opposite sex

2. _____ Individuals who are attracted to both sexes

3. _____ Individuals who are attracted to the same sex

4. _____ Individuals who are not particularly attracted to either sex

5. _____ Women who are sexually attracted to women

6. _____ Men who are sexually attracted to men

Column II

a. Bisexual

b. Homosexual

c. Asexual

d. Gay

e. Heterosexual

f. Lesbian

Part 5

Indicate if the following action would be appropriate (A) or inappropriate (I).

1. _____ Explaining to a woman that chlamydia is the involuntary contraction of vaginal outlet muscles that prevents penile penetration

2. _____ Explaining to a man that a vasectomy is an ideal form of birth control because it can be reversed if he should want children at some later time

3. _____ Cautioning sexually active teens that although many sexually transmitted diseases (STDs) are treatable, there are antibiotic-resistant organisms and organisms no treatment can cure

4. _____ Monitoring for a chancre on the penis or vagina of a client as a sign of syphilis

5. _____ Teaching clients with herpes simplex virus 2 that they must complete 2 weeks of antibiotics to completely cure the infection

Part 6 Short Answer Exercises

Complete the following by filling in the blanks.

1. The sexual response cycle is divided into _____, _____, _____, and resolution.

2. When assisting a couple in choosing a method of birth control, the nurse should consider _____, _____, and _____.

3. Briefly define three hormonal methods of birth control. _____

4. Methods of birth control include hormonal, _____ devices, _____ methods, natural methods, and _____ of the man, woman, or both partners.

70

Fundamentals of Pediatric Nursing

Common Acronyms or Terms

DtP

I & O

IV

LP

MMR

NPO

OFC

PICC

TPN

URI

CHAPTER OVERVIEW

Chapter 70 discusses the care of the pediatric client. Concerns related to health maintenance, hospitalization, and basic assessment, treatment, and discharge procedures are addressed. The nurse's role in helping the child and family to meet the basic needs of the child is explored.

✪ Be sure to review the Learning Objectives from the text.

✎ Be sure to FIRST perform Improving Concentration exercises described in the Introduction before proceeding with the next exercise.

Part 1

Indicate in which order the following major headings would be found in this chapter.

1. _____ Health Maintenance
2. _____ Meeting Basic Needs
3. _____ The Child Having Surgery
4. _____ The Hospital Experience
5. _____ Basic Pediatric Problems
6. _____ Advanced Pediatric Procedures

Part 2

Complete the following statements related to the major headings and key points.

1. The major heading The Hospital Experience contains subheadings that address: _____-_____ concerns, _____-centered care, and _____.

2. _____ is children's work and their means of communication.

3. Pediatrics requires knowledge of developmental _____; this knowledge helps you determine developmental _____.

4. Very _____ children are especially susceptible to communicable diseases.

Part 3 Key Terms: Knowledge Check

Review the key terms in the chapter. Unscramble the letters to reveal the terms that match the definitions provided.

1. Ascepritid _____
   Area of care that deals with children and adolescents

2. Manimuzitoni _____
   Provides people with temporary or permanent protection against certain diseases

3. Inetapiridac _____
   Provider in the field of care that deals with children

Part 4

Match the sites for vital signs listed in column I with the appropriate age range in column II.

Column I

1. _____ Radial pulse

2. _____ Oral or tympanic temperature

3. _____ Use an infant scale

4. _____ Measure head circumference

5. _____ Record standing height

Column II

a. Children older than 6 years of age

b. Children up to 3 years of age

c. Older children

d. Children older than 2 years of age

e. Small children

Part 5 Short Answer and Completions

Complete the following by filling in the blanks.

1. Children may need _____ to remind them not to pull on tubes or pick at suture lines; these should be removed and reapplied every _____ to _____ hours and the child's skin and circulation checked _____ hour.

2. _____ substitute the safety device for good observation.

3. Early immunization is important to _____ small children.

4. Identify the appropriate age range in which the following immunizations should be administered:

   a. _____ Hep B-1

   b. _____ Polio

   c. _____ Hib

   d. _____ Measles, mumps, rubella

   e. _____ Diphtheria, tetanus, pertussis

5. List four signs of respiratory distress in a child

   _____

   _____

   _____

   _____

Part 6 Multiple Choice Exercises

Circle the letter corresponding to the correct answer.

1. Lela Morales, age 3, is admitted with abdominal pain. She has an order to have a urine culture. Which of the following accurately describes a step in collecting a urine specimen?
   a. Tell Lela to lie on her stomach with a bedpan under her perineum.
   b. Clean Lela's perineal area adding powder to the thighs and labia to protect them from urine.
   c. Apply a urine collector to Lela's perineum sealing from the bottom up to the pubis.
   d. Cover the bag with a tight-fitting diaper or underpants to hold it in place.

2. You assess that Lela, your 3-year-old client, is restless and apprehensive and has nasal flaring and tachypnea. You would:
   a. Recognize that Lela needs comfort and pick her up in your arms and rock her gently
   b. Acknowledge the signs that Lela is in respiratory distress and prepare to give oxygen by mist tent or oxyhood
   c. Determine that this is not unusual behavior for a 3-year-old, and would ask the parents or guardian to sit with her
   d. Offer Lela a special treat if she would calm down, then give her candy and praise her for cooperating

3. You need to give Lela, 3 years old, a liquid medication. She refused the medication on the previous shift by spitting it out each time given. You could do which of the following?
   a. Tell Lela firmly that she must take the medication and that crying will not be tolerated.
   b. Give Lela a drop or two of the liquid over about an hour to prevent spitting it out.
   c. Tell Lela the medicine is a sweet candy syrup that she will like.
   d. Be positive and ask Lela if she would like to take her medication from a cup or spoon.

4. Lela, 3 years old, is scheduled for abdominal exploratory surgery. Which of the following would be appropriate in preoperative or postoperative care for Lela?

a. Check for voiding, postoperatively, and if permitted, offer to help her to the bathroom/potty to void.

b. Encourage Lela, postoperatively, to move her hands, fingers, and arms to prevent thrombophlebitis.

c. Have Lela sign the operative permit form with the mother cosigning; the student nurse should sign as witness for both signatures.

d. Dress Lela in her favorite pajamas so she will feel secure and as if she were going to sleep.

71

Care of the Infant, Toddler, or Preschooler

Common Acronyms or Terms

ALL	LOC
AML	LTB
ASO	MMR
AV	MRI
BRAT	MTX
CF	NPO
CNS	O & P
CPR	OFC
CPT	ORS
CT	PDA
DH	PE
DtP	PKU
ECG	PET
ED	PIA
EEG	RBC
ESR	RSV
FTT	SGA
GI	SIDS
HUS	T&A
I & O	TPN
ITP	URI
IV	WBC

CHAPTER OVERVIEW

Chapter 71 discusses disorders common to children who are infant to preschool age. Nursing care for children in this age range is addressed.

✪ Be sure to review the Learning Objectives from the text.

✔ Be sure to FIRST perform Improving Concentration exercises described in the Introduction before proceeding with the next exercise.

Part 1

Complete the following titles of major headings and statements related to the key points.

1. T_____

2. Disorders of the E_____

3. N_____ Disorders

4. S_____ Disorders

5. C_____ Diseases

6. The major heading that contains subheadings on Marasmus, and Biliary Atresia is M_____ and N_____ Disorders.

7. Many childhood communicable diseases can be prevented through _____.

8. _____ of _____ exists in more than 90% of all near-drowning events.

9. Illness of the GI tract places the young child at high risk for _____ and _____ imbalance or _____.

10. _____, the most serious form of spina bifida, may cause paralysis or other disorders.

Part 2 Key Terms: Knowledge Check

Answer these statements true (T) or false (F).

1. _____ Bronchiolitis is a viral respiratory infection resulting in inflammation of the bronchioles.

2. _____ Encopresis is the telescoping of one bowel part into another.

3. _____ Cryptorchidism is an undescended testicle.

4. _____ Intussusception is the incontinence of feces without physical cause.

5. _____ Rickets, also called wryneck, in the congenital form is caused by failure of the sternocleidomastoid muscle to lengthen as the child grows.

Part 3

Fill in the term or terms that best match(es) the definition.

1. _____
   If the bones in the fetal skull do not close correctly, a portion of the brain may herniate through the opening.

2. _____
   General failure to thrive (FTT)

3. _____
   Involves small bowel inflammation and nutrient malabsorption

4. _____
   Acute and potentially fatal childhood disease with fever, cerebral edema, impaired liver function, and severely impaired LOC; usually follows a viral illness and aspirin use

Part 4

Match the statement in column I with the closely related term or concept in column II.

Column I

1. _____ Describes a foot that is twisted or bent out of shape as a result of hereditary factors or an abnormal fetal position; treated with casting or splinting to correct the deformity

2. _____ Common measles, red measles; caused by a virus found in the nose, mouth, throat, eyes, and their discharges; highly communicable

3. _____ A benign disease of infancy in which a high fever is followed by a rash appearing on the trunk then spreading to the neck, face, and extremities when the child's temperature falls

4. _____ A viral infection that is mild but can cause serious fetal malformations if a pregnant woman contracts the disease; German measles

5. _____ A child's colon lacking parasympathetic nerve supply resulting in lack of peristalsis

6. _____ A group of associated disorders characterized by malignancies in the bone marrow and lymphatic system

Column II

a. Rubeola

b. Leukemia

c. Hirschsprung's disease

d. Talipes

e. Roseola

f. Rubella

Part 5

Indicate if the following actions are appropriate (A) or inappropriate (I).

1. ____ Providing a child with celiac disease a diet with carbohydrates supplied by wheat and barley

2. ____ Administering acetaminophen and tepid sponge baths to a child experiencing febrile seizures

3. ____ Placing elbow restraints on a child after surgery for correction of strabismus

4. ____ Feeding a child with cleft lip and palate using a cup and straw to promote independence

5. ____ Using the side of a spoon to feed a child after cleft palate repair

6. ____ Teaching parents of an infant being monitored for apnea to stimulate the child immediately if the monitor alarms even if the child is pink

7. ____ When a child informs you that his uncle is sexually abusing him, you should consider the age of the child and say nothing because young children are easily confused.

8. ____ Attempting to establish a supportive relationship with the caregivers of a suspected child abuse victim

Part 6 Labeling Exercise

Indicate the name of the defects in tetralogy of Fallot marked with lines in the illustration below.

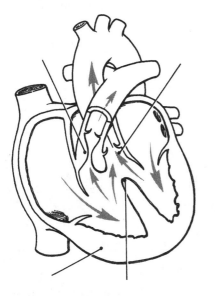

Part 7

1. Ben Tashah, age 6, is suspected of having tetralogy of Fallot. Which of the following symptoms would *not* assist in confirming this diagnosis:
   a. Cyanosis
   b. Signs of hypoxia
   c. History that Ben often squats when he is out of breath
   d. A fine red rash noted on Ben's chest and legs
2. Vicki Tee, 10 years old, has asthma. She was admitted in acute distress last week and is being discharged home. The nurse should review which of the following with Vicki and her parents?
   a. The benefits of pet therapy in helping Vicki relax; rubbing on her cat or dog during an acute episode of asthma may calm her and help her breathing
   b. That medications to treat asthma should be taken when the asthma attack has fully begun to maximize the effectiveness of the medication
   c. The need for Vicki to use the peak flow meter and to keep a diary of the peak flow and asthma symptoms
   d. The use of epinephrine daily to prevent an asthma attack and the need to take medications over a long period, not just on an as needed basis

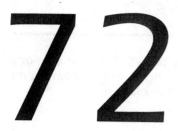

Care of the School-Age Child or Adolescent

Common Acronyms or Terms

AN

CUC

IBD

IDDM

JRA

NSAID

REM

RP

STD

CHAPTER OVERVIEW

Chapter 72 discusses disorders common to children who are school-age to adolescent age. Nursing care for children in this age range is addressed.

✪ Be sure to review the Learning Objectives from the text.

✔ Be sure to FIRST perform Improving Concentration exercises described in the Introduction before proceeding with the next exercise.

Part 1

Complete the following titles of major headings and statements related to the key points in this chapter.

1. C_____ Diseases

2. R_____
   S_____ Disorders

3. G _____ Disorders

4. S____ Disorders

5. M_____ Disorders

6. The major heading that contains a subheading on Diabetes Mellitus is E_____ Disorders.

7. _____ Nervosa and _____, although related to nutrition, are psychological disorders requiring long-term treatment.

8. Hormonal changes occurring in the older child result in certain disorders, including _____ vulgaris, _____ difficulties, and _____ disorders.

Part 2 Key Terms: Knowledge Check

Review the key terms in the chapter. Correct the following definitions by supplying the correct key term. Hint: all the terms are present, just mixed with the wrong definition.

1. _____ *Hypersomnia* is characterized by a progressive bilateral retinal degeneration that often causes blindness.

2. _____ *Impetigo* contagiosa is an attack of muscle weakness and lack of muscle tone; may accompany narcolepsy.

3. _____ *Retinitis* pigmentosa is sleep walking; usually occurs during the later stages of non-REM sleep.

4. _____ *Somnambulism* is pain occurring with ovulation.

5. _____ *Mittelschmerz* is an uncontrolled urge to sleep; lengthy sleep periods of 12 to 18 hours.

6. _____ *Cataplexy* is an infection caused by staphylococci or mixed bacteria; usually vesicles break out on the face and hands.

Part 3

Fill in the term or terms that best match(es) the definition.

1. _____
   Brief attack of irresistible sleep; conflict, competition, and unacceptable aggression may be underlying contributing factors.

2. _____
   A self-limiting disease characterized by flu-like symptoms and caused by the Epstein-Barr virus

3. _____
   Refers to faulty tooth positioning, which results in improper alignment of the jaws and teeth

4. _____
   Correction of tooth positioning and jaw deformities

Part 4

Match the statement in column I with the closely related term or concept in column II.

Column I

1. _____ Painful menstruation; the nurse might administer acetaminophen or ibuprofen for relief.

2. _____ Sleep talking; the person may carry on a logical conversation but not remember it the next morning.

3. _____ A tick-borne illness; person may develop a ring-shaped rash, and flulike symptoms that progress to angina, limb numbness, loss of muscle function and a diversity of symptoms.

4. _____ A surgical means of smoothing the skin; may be considered after active acne has ceased.

5. _____ This eating disorder is characterized by binge eating, followed by purging.

Column II

a. Bulimia

b. Somniloquism

c. Dermabrasion

d. Lyme disease

e. Dysmenorrhea

Part 5

Indicate if the following actions are appropriate (A) or inappropriate (I).

1. _____ Instructing a teen with acne to use gentle cleaning and to avoid scrubbing the face

2. _____ Suggesting that young people wear sandals and cotton socks if they have athlete's foot

3. _____ Keeping a child with Legg-Calvé-Perthes disease physically active to build the muscles in the legs

4. _____ Administering nonsteroidal anti-inflammatory drugs (NSAIDs) and hot baths to a child with juvenile rheumatoid arthritis

5. _____ Instructing a child with retinitis pigmentosa that sunglasses or shades should be avoided to prevent sensory deprivation to eyes

6. _____ Preparing to administer steroids to a teen with inflammatory bowel disease

7. _____ Informing the parents of a child who experiences night terrors that noting spots of blood after an episode is expected and nothing to worry about

8. _____ Assisting the family of a youngster who is a chronic lawbreaker in arranging for family counseling

Part 6 Labeling Exercise

*Indicate which picture demonstrates the spinal deviation in **A—scoliosis, B—kyphosis, C—lordosis, D—normal (one letter will not be used).***

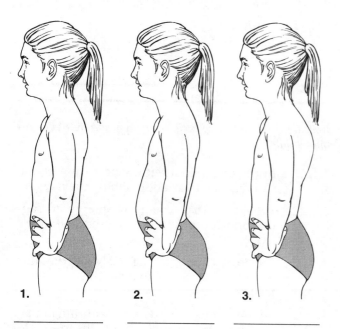

1. _____

2. _____

3. _____

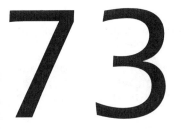

_____ Mental Illness

_____ Long-Term Care

_____ Learning Disabilities

_____ Chronic Lead Poisoning (Plumbism)

_____ Sensory Disorders

The Child or Adolescent With Special Needs

Common Acronyms or Terms

ADDH	COA	II
ADHD	CP	IQ
ADL	CPK	MBD
AFP	EEG	MD
AIDS	FAS	SLD
ALT	FTT	
CNS	HIV	

CHAPTER OVERVIEW

Chapter 73 discusses the concerns and care of the child with special needs. An overview of various conditions that alter intellectual, emotional, and physical growth and development is provided.

✪ Be sure to review the Learning Objectives from the text.

✔ Be sure to FIRST perform Improving Concentration exercises described in the Introduction before proceeding with the next exercise.

Part 1

Indicate the order in which you find the following major headings in this chapter.

Part 2

Complete the following statements related to the major headings and key points.

1. Maternal use of _____ or _____ can result in physical or mental abnormalities in a newborn.

2. The two subheadings found in this chapter under Long-Term Neuromuscular Disorders are _____ _____ and _____ _____ _____.

3. A common finding in children with learning disabilities is low _____ _____.

4. Caregivers of a child with special needs may grieve over the loss of the _____ _____.

Part 3 Key Terms: Knowledge Check

Unscramble the letters to identify the term that best matches the definition.

1. Tusaim _____
   Severe developmental disorder characterized by intellectual, social, and communication deficits

2. Icudise _____
   Inflicting personal injury with intent to cause death; third leading cause of death in 15- to 19-year-old adolescents

3. Fenuclydsy _____
   Interruption in the natural flow of speaking

4. Axiledsy _____
   Disorder in which the person has difficulty reading, spelling, or writing words

Part 4

Indicate if these nursing actions would be appropriate (A) or inappropriate (I).

1. _____ Instructing the parents of a child with AIDS that immunizations and isolation from other sick children are critical

2. _____ Using IQ scores to determine a child's abilities and plan education

3. _____ Focusing nursing interventions for the child with Down syndrome on treatments to increase the child's IQ scores with age

4. _____ When caring for a child with a specific learning disability (SLD), learning about the specific disability and setting achievable goals

5. _____ Providing a child with visual processing deficits with a tape recorder that reinforces information

6. _____ Teaching family caregivers of a child with attention deficit-hyperactivity disorder to increase environmental stimuli to overcome the deficit

7. _____ Keeping the child with plumbism in the home and teaching him or her not to eat the paint in the home or play with other items that contain lead

8. _____ Helping the child with cerebral palsy learn self-care activities

Part 5

Match the concepts and definitions in column I with the classifications or title in column II.

Column I

1. _____ The most common case of cerebral palsy, symptoms include hypertension and increased stretch reflexes.

2. _____ A form of cerebral palsy that occurs in 20% of cases; characterized by abnormal involuntary movements such as grimacing and sharp jerks.

3. _____ A cognitively impaired child with an IQ of 36 to 51; achieves a maximum mental age of 3 to 7 years.

4. _____ A cognitively impaired child who requires complete assistance with all aspects of daily life; IQ below 19 (unable to test)

5. _____ Person loses contact with reality; sometimes results from a sudden, severe emotional experience and familial tendencies have been noted.

Column II

a. Spastic cerebral palsy

b. Schizophrenic

c. Moderate cognitive impairment

d. Dyskinetic cerebral palsy

e. Profound cognitive impairment

Part 6 Short Answer Exercises

Complete the following statements by filling in the blanks.

1. A _____ disorder is a physical or mental abnormality resulting from a defect in genetic structure, whereas a _____ disorder occurs due to contact a pregnant woman has with teratogens.

2. Compare Down syndrome and fragile X syndrome relative to head, face, and ears. _____

_____

_____

3. What measures should a nurse take when assisting a child with long-term disability? _____

_____

_____

74

Skin Disorders

Common Acronyms or Terms

AgNO$_3$

CEA

DTIC

I & O

IV

mL/kg

mm Hg

PRN

ROM

SPF

TBSA

TPN

UV

CHAPTER OVERVIEW

Chapter 74 gives an overview of common skin disorders and discusses their relationships with the body system primarily involved with the condition.

✪ Be sure to review the Learning Objectives from the text.

✔ Be sure to FIRST perform Improving Concentration exercises described in the Introduction before proceeding with the next exercise.

Part 1 Multiple Choice

Circle the letter corresponding to the correct answer based on the location in the topics outline.

1. An example of a sebaceous gland disorder would be:
   a. Dermatitis
   b. Eczema
   c. Warts
   d. Scabies

2. Nonmalignant tumors are considered:
   a. Parasitic infestations
   b. Sebaceous gland disorders
   c. Acute and chronic skin conditions
   d. Neoplasms

3. Urticaria is considered to be in the category of:
   a. Sebaceous gland disorders
   b. Neoplasms
   c. Acute and chronic skin conditions
   d. Infections

4. Skin and tissue grafts can be researched under the heading of:
   a. Burns
   b. Common surgical treatments
   c. Common medical treatments
   d. Neoplasms

5. Information on warts will be found in the heading of:
   a. Neoplasms
   b. Common medical treatments
   c. Infections
   d. Acute and chronic skin conditions

Part 2

Based on information found in the key points, complete the following sentences.

1. Wood's light examination and tissue biopsy are examples of common _____ tests.

2. _____ and _____ are common bacterial skin infections.

3. Autografts and allografts are two examples of major types of _____.

4. Various allergies may cause urticaria and _____.

5. _____ is the study of skin diseases.

6. The four types of burns are thermal, _____, chemical, and _____.

7. The integumentary system is composed of the _____ and its accessory organs.

8. Moles, _____, and keloids are examples of _____ skin tumors.

9. Scabies, lice, and bedbugs are examples of _____ skin infestations.

10. Malignant melanoma is a type of skin _____.

Part 3 Key Terms: Knowledge Check

Review the key terms and change one word in each sentence to make it true.

1. Eschar is viable skin and tissue that sloughs off following a burn.
2. Angioedema is a life-threatening condition similar to urticaria but involves superficial dermal and subcutaneous tissues.
3. When a person's own skin can be used this is considered a homograft.
4. Vitiligo is a disorder in which areas of the skin are partially lacking in pigmentation.
5. Cyrosurgery involves the application of liquid hydrogen.
6. Impetigo is commonly caused by a streptococcal or staphylococcal virus and is contagious.
7. A xenograft involves the grafting of cadaver skin in some severe burns.
8. Contractures result from the abnormal lengthening of muscles, tendons, or scar tissue.
9. Psoriasis is a chronic, contagious, proliferative skin disorder.
10. Condylomata acuminata are also called venereal keloids.

Part 4 Clinical Thinking

You are assisting with the care of Mr. Gaston Jones, a 36-year-old firefighter who is admitted for burn injuries. Answer the questions based on the information found under the heading of burns.

1. Mr. Jones will have his burns evaluated and classified as either _____ or full thickness.

2. He may undergo an escharotomy if he has sustained any circumferential burns to restore _____ functions or ease of _____.

3. The three phases of burn injury management are _____, acute, and _____.

4. Black or gray sputum may indicate _____.

5. The leading cause of death for people with burns is _____.

75

Disorders in Fluid and Electrolyte Balance

Common Acronyms or Terms

C	ICF	mg/dL
Ca	I & O	Na
CNS	IV	P
CO_2	K	pH
ECF	mEq/L	PO_4
GI	Mg	

CHAPTER OVERVIEW

Chapter 75 discusses the importance of maintaining homeostasis and the effect of disorders in various body systems on the normal balance of the body's fluids and electrolytes.

✪ Be sure to review the Learning Objectives from the text.

✔ Be sure to FIRST perform Improving Concentration exercises described in the Introduction before proceeding with the next exercise.

Part 1

Answer these statements true (T) or false (F) based on a review of the major headings and key points. Correct the false.

1. _____ Edematous skin is friable and prone to breakdown.

2. _____ Measurement of I & O and hourly weights is an important component in the assessment of fluid balance.

3. _____ Respiratory acidosis, if not corrected, could lead to the need for mechanical ventilation.

4. _____ Information on edema can be found under the heading Maintenance of Electrolyte Balance.

5. _____ Fluid and electrolyte disturbances can occur in anyone.

Part 2 The Numbers Game

Fill in the blanks using the list of numbers provided.

1. Hyperkalemia means a serum potassium level of

   _____.

2. Water comprises up to _____%
   of the human body.

3. Extracellular fluid (ECF) is normally maintained at
   a pH of approximately _____.

4. Hyponatremia means a serum sodium level of less
   than _____.

5. Clients with fluid volume deficits should have
   good mouth care performed every _____ hours.

   75

   5.5

   2

   7.4

   135

Part 3 Key Terms: Knowledge Check

Circle the letter corresponding to the correct answer based on knowledge of the key terms.

1. A deficit in bicarbonate ions or an excess of hydrogen ions causes a condition called:
   a. Metabolic alkalosis
   b. Metabolic acidosis
   c. Respiratory alkalosis
   d. Respiratory acidosis

2. Overhydration refers specially to excess water in the:
   a. Intracellular spaces
   b. Interstitial spaces
   c. Extracellular spaces
   d. Extrathecal spaces

3. A dent that remains for some time after edematous tissue over a bone is pressed with a finger is called _____ edema.
   a. Dependent
   b. Sacral
   c. Pitting
   d. Pulmonary

4. A deficit of plasma CO_2 or carbonic acid results in a condition called:
   a. Metabolic alkalosis
   b. Metabolic acidosis
   c. Respiratory alkalosis
   d. Respiratory acidosis

5. The term ascites describes the accumulation of fluid in the:
   a. Abdominal cavity
   b. Interstitial spaces
   c. Renal pelvis
   d. Lower extremities

76

Musculoskeletal Disorders

Common Acronyms or Terms

AEA	IVD
AKA	LD
AS	NSAID
BEA	ORIF
BKA	PCA
CK	RA
CMS	RF
CPM	ROM
DJD	SLE
DVT	TENS
EF	THA
EMG	TLSO
ESR	TMJ

CHAPTER OVERVIEW

Chapter 76 reviews the anatomy and physiology of the musculoskeletal system and discusses the most common disease states.

✪ Be sure to review the Learning Objectives from the text.

✔ Be sure to FIRST perform Improving Concentration exercises described in the Introduction before proceeding with the next exercise.

Part 1

Match the subheadings in column I with the headings in column II. Some letters will be used more than once.

Column I

1. Fractures
2. Gout
3. Evaluation
4. Arthroplasty
5. Hemorrhage
6. Chronic Back Pain
7. Rickets
8. Traction
9. X-Ray Evaluations
10. Data Collection
11. Deep Vein Thrombosis
12. Amputation
13. Internal Fixation
14. Casts
15. Laboratory Tests

Column II

A. Common Medical Treatments
B. Nursing Process
C. Musculoskeletal Disorders
D. Diagnostic Tests
E. Complications Related to Musculoskeletal Disorders
F. Trauma
G. Common Surgical Techniques
H. Systemic Disorders With Musculoskeletal Manifestations

Part 2

Based on a review of the key points, change one word to make the sentence true.

1. Malignant bone tumors grow slowly and rarely spread.
2. A cast stabilizes and mobilizes fractures.
3. Try to prevent complications caused by a client's increased mobility.
4. In skeletal traction the pull is applied to the skin.
5. Sprains and strains are examples of nontraumatic injuries.

Part 3 Key Terms: Knowledge Check

Supply the correct term for each definition below.

1. _____
   Repair or replacement of a joint

2. _____
   Artificial device that replaces part or all of a missing extremity

3. _____
   Loosening of dead bone fragments

4. _____
   Joint inflammation

5. _____
   Inflammation of the tendon sheath

6. _____
   Invasive procedure that allows endoscopic examination of various joints

7. _____
   Serious bone infection that is curable if detected and treated appropriately

8. _____
   Calcification of joint so that movement is impossible

9. _____
   Collagen disorder; the term means "hard skin."

10. _____
    Displacement of a bone from its socket

Part 4 Multiple Choice

Circle the letter corresponding to the correct answer.

1. The most painful and crippling form of arthritis is:
   a. Osteoarthritis
   b. Rheumatoid arthritis
   c. Ankylosing spondylitis
   d. Degenerative joint disease

2. An x-ray examination of the spinal cord and vertebral canal after the injection of contrast medium or air into the spinal subarachnoid space is called a:
   a. CT scan
   b. MRI
   c. Myelogram
   d. Electromyogram

3. Inflammation of the fluid-filled sac that pads the bony prominences in the joints is called:
   a. Tenosynovitis
   b. Bursitis
   c. Epicondylitis
   d. Arthritis

4. All the statements concerning compartment syndrome are true EXCEPT:
   a. Permanent muscle and nerve damage can result in 4 to 6 days if uncorrected.
   b. Contractures may develop.
   c. The cardinal symptom is pain unrelieved by medications and aggravated by passive stretching of the ischemic muscle.
   d. It is a medical emergency.

5. Gout is the result of the inability of the body to metabolize purines resulting in the accumulation of:
   a. Gastric acid
   b. Acetic acid
   c. Hydrochloric acid
   d. Uric acid

Part 5 Clinical Thinking

You admit Mrs. Petrovich to your unit after application of a halo device. You have to decide where to place the wrench. Explain where you place the wrench.

_____

_____

77

Nervous System Disorders

Common Acronyms or Terms

ADL

ALS

ATM

CHT

CNS

CSF

CT

EEG

HD

HZ

ICP

IICP

LOC

LP

MAO

MG

MRI

MS

PD

PET

SE

TPN

CHAPTER OVERVIEW

Chapter 77 reviews the anatomy and physiology of the nervous system, common treatments, the nursing process, and various disorders common to the nervous system.

✪ Be sure to review the Learning Objectives from the text.

✔ Be sure to FIRST perform Improving Concentration exercises described in the Introduction before proceeding with the next exercise.

Part 1

Identify the heading under which you would find the following information.

1. Carpal tunnel syndrome _____

2. Hematoma _____

3. Evaluation _____

4. Multiple sclerosis _____

5. Guillian-Barré syndrome _____

6. Concussion _____

7. Meningitis _____

8. Parkinson's disease _____

9. Shingles _____

10. Headache _____

Part 2

Based on the major headings and key points, complete the following sentences by filling in the blanks.

1. Inflammatory disorders of the nervous system can

   quickly become _____ - _____.

2. Seizure disorders are located under the heading

   _____

   _____.

3. One of the first and most important signs of IICP is

   a change in the _____.

4. Most brain tumors are _____.

5. An example of a common surgical treatment is a

   _____

   _____.

Part 3 Key Terms: Knowledge Check

Answer these statements true (T) or false (F). Correct the false.

1. _____ Quadriplegia means paralysis of all four extremities.

2. _____ Intracranial pressure (ICP) is the pressure that the brain, blood, and CSF exert outside the cerebrospinal cavity.

3. _____ Neuralgia literally means pain in a nerve.

4. _____ Ataxia refers to a condition characterized by defective nerve coordination.

5. _____ Meningitis is an inflammation limited to the membranes surrounding the brain.

6. _____ Autonomic dysreflexia is also known as a sudden, dangerous high blood sugar.

7. _____ A hematoma is the result of any blow to the head.

8. _____ A craniotomy is a noninvasive procedure.

9. _____ Cephalalgia is also commonly known as myelitis.

10. _____ A seizure is a result of an abnormal discharge of neurons in the brain.

Part 4

Choose the disease in column II that matches the most with the associated symptoms outlined in column I.

Column I

1. _____ Onset is sudden.

2. _____ Muscle weakness can lead to total paralysis.

3. _____ Begins in lower extremities and ascends.

4. _____ Recovery is slow.

5. _____ Emotional support is essential.

6. _____ Excellent nursing care is necessary.

7. _____ Recovery is often complete.

Column II

a. Multiple sclerosis

b. Guillian-Barré disease

c. Parkinson's disease

78

Endocrine Disorders

Common Acronyms or Terms

ACE	IFG
ACTH	IGT
ADA	LH
ADH	NHS
BIDS	NIDDM
BR	OGTT
FPG	PTH
FSH	RAIU
GDM	SIADH
GH	SMBG
GSH	STH
GTT	TFT
I & O	TSH
IDDM	VMA

CHAPTER OVERVIEW

Chapter 78 reviews the anatomy and physiology of the endocrine system and describes common diagnostic tests used in the evaluation of endocrine disorders.

✪ Be sure to review the Learning Objectives from the text.

✔ Be sure to FIRST perform Improving Concentration exercises described in the Introduction before proceeding with the next exercise.

Part 1 Multiple Choice

Using information from the headings and key points, circle the letter corresponding to the correct answer.

1. Diabetes mellitus occurs when either the body becomes resistant to or this organ does not make enough insulin.
   a. Thyroid
   b. Pituitary
   c. Pancreas
   d. Adrenal

2. Goiter is categorized as a disorder of the:
   a. Pituitary
   b. Thyroid
   c. Parathyroid
   d. Adrenal gland

3. A serum ACTH test would be found under the category:
   a. Pituitary function tests
   b. Thyroid function tests
   c. Adrenal function tests
   d. General pancreatic function tests

4. Hypophysectomy is considered a:
   a. Common medical treatment
   b. Common surgical treatment
   c. Thyroid disorder
   d. Parathyroid disorder

5. Serum amylase would be found under the category:
   a. Pituitary function tests
   b. Thyroid function tests
   c. Adrenal function tests
   d. General pancreatic function tests

Part 2 Key Terms: Knowledge Check

Using the words from the Key Terms list, supply the correct term for the definitions below.

1. _____
   Decreased tissue sensitivity to insulin

2. _____
   Condition in adults resulting from an excess of somatotropin, which causes an overgrowth of tissues

3. _____
   Catecholamine-secreting adrenal tumor

4. _____
   May be positive with low calcium level characterized by an abnormal spasm of the facial muscles in response to light taps on the facial nerve

5. _____
   Condition resulting from overproduction of the hormones secreted by the adrenal cortex. Fat distribution is abnormal.

Part 3

Using words from the key terms, complete the terms.

1. Poly_____: excessive thirst
2. Hyper_____: abnormally high blood sugar
3. Poly_____: excessive hunger
4. Hypo_____: also called myxedema
5. Hypo_____: surgical removal of the pituitary
6. Hyper_____: stems from an excess of PTH, which causes an elevated calcium level in the blood
7. Poly_____: excessive urination

Part 4 Clinical Thinking

Choose the best answer from the choices provided after reading the following scenario.

You are taking vital signs on Mrs. Stone who has recently been diagnosed with Graves' disease. You note that her pulse is rapid, her systolic blood pressure is elevated, and her eyes appear to be bulging. You are:
1. Alarmed because these symptoms are not consistent with her diagnosis
2. Concerned when you read the term exophthalmos documented on her chart because that term is not associated with Graves' disease
3. Anxious to report these new findings to your charge nurse
4. Aware that these symptoms are consistent with the diagnosis of Graves' disease

Part 5

Using information found in the heading Diabetes Mellitus, under what subheading would you find the following information?

1. Type I versus type II _____
2. Goals of diabetes management _____
3. Hypoglycemic reaction _____
4. Polyphagia _____
5. Foot care _____
6. Insulin resistance _____
7. Identification _____
8. Exercise _____
9. Numbness and tingling in extremities _____
_____
10. Ketoacidosis _____

79

Sensory System Disorders

Common Acronyms or Terms

EEG	OD
ENG	OS
ERG	OSHA
IOL	OU
MRI	RGP

CHAPTER OVERVIEW

Chapter 79 reviews the anatomy and physiology of the sensory system and discusses common medical and surgical treatments, common disorders, and diagnostic tests.

✪ Be sure to review the Learning Objectives from the text.

✔ Be sure to FIRST perform Improving Concentration exercises described in the Introduction before proceeding with the next exercise.

Part 1

Using information from the headings and key points, change one word to make the sentence true.

1. Refractive disorders result when light rays focus improperly on the iris.
2. Refraction is the required treatment for cataracts.
3. Most eye and ear surgeries are done on an inpatient basis using the operating microscope.

4. Eye and vision disorders include inflammatory and noninfectious disorders.
5. Hearing deficits are caused by diseases, congenital, and nonenvironmental factors.

Part 2 Key Terms: Knowledge Check

Using the list of words from the key terms, circle the letter corresponding to the correct answer.

1. The procedure in which the eyeball is removed is called:
   a. Ectropion
   b. Entropion
   c. Enucleation
   d. Ptosis

2. The contagious inflammation of the membrane lining the eyelids and covering the sclera is:
   a. Blepharitis
   b. Conjunctivitis
   c. Tinnitus
   d. Otosclerosis

3. The term to describe an accumulation of lipid material from a chronically obstructed meibomian gland is:
   a. Chalazion
   b. Ectropion
   c. Entropion
   d. Hyphema

4. This procedure involves the plastic reconstruction of the tiny bones of the middle ear.
   a. Keratoplasty
   b. Myringotomy
   c. Tympanoplasty
   d. Hyphema

5. The medical term for ringing in the ears is:
   a. Conjunctivitis
   b. Tinnitus
   c. Ptosis
   d. Otosclerosis

Part 3 Clinical Thinking

As an optometric nurse for Dr. Meniere you have administered eye drops to dilate the client's pupils before an examination by the doctor. Mrs. Hale suddenly complains of blurred vision, a halo around the ceiling light, severe pain in her eye, and feeling nauseous. You recognize the symptoms of:

a. Meniere's disease
b. Open-angle glaucoma
c. Narrow-angle glaucoma
d. Detached retina

80

Cardiovascular Disorders

Common Acronyms or Terms

AICD	CPR	NS
AST	CVA	PE
BP	DVT	PROM
CAD	ECG	PT
CC	EPS	PTCA
CCU	HTN	PTT
CHF	I & O	t-PA
CICU	ICD	TPN
CPK	LDH	VV
CPM	MI	

CHAPTER OVERVIEW

Chapter 80 reviews the anatomy and physiology of the cardiovascular system and discusses diagnostic tests, common medical and surgical treatments, and disorders common to the cardiovascular system.

✪ Be sure to review the Learning Objectives from the text.

✔ Be sure to FIRST perform Improving Concentration exercises described in the Introduction before proceeding with the next exercise.

Part 1

Determine the heading of the topics outline that contains information about the following subheadings.

1. _____ Aneurysms
2. _____ Thrombolytic therapy
3. _____ PCTA
4. _____ Coronary artery disease
5. _____ CVA

Part 2

Using information from the key points, answer the following questions by changing one word to make the statement true.

1. Hearing and vision are usually impaired on the nonaffected side after a CVA.
2. Angina or angina pectoris is a permanent loss of oxygen to the heart muscle.
3. All types of heart disease can be cured.
4. Hypertension will lead to serious problems such as myocardial infarction, kidney damage, congestive heart failure, and cerebrovascular accident.
5. Death of heart tissue is called myocardial ischemia.

Part 3 Nursing Alert

Complete the following statements based on information found in the nursing alerts located throughout the chapter.

1. You are taking the first set of vital signs of a client who has returned to your unit after a cardiac catheterization. You note that his pulse is rapid and irregular compared to his pulse before the procedure. You realize that this may indicate heart or _____ damage, clot formation or _____.

2. If a client with a pacemaker notices any symptoms of _____ or light-headedness instruct him or her to move at least _____ feet from the source of any _____ interference.

3. Angina pain that lasts more than _____ minutes is considered an MI until proven otherwise.

4. To avoid having to repeat what you say and perhaps embarrassing the person who has experienced a CVA, the nurse should approach the person from the _____ side.

5. Ask clients if they are allergic to _____ or _____ before performing any test in which radiopaque dye is used.

Part 4

Using words from the key terms, match the terms in column I with the definitions in column II.

Column I

1. _____ Aphasia
2. _____ Myocarditis
3. _____ Myocardial infarction
4. _____ Fibrillation
5. _____ Stent
6. _____ Angioplasty
7. _____ Endocarditis

Column II

a. Disorganized twitching of cardiac muscle

b. Inflammation of heart's inner lining

c. Procedure to widen the lumen of an artery

d. Inability to speak

e. Inflammation of the heart's muscular walls

f. Heart attack

g. Wire coil used to keep an artery open

81

NHL
PBSC
PPF
PT
PTT
RBC
T & C
WBC

Blood and Lymph Disorders

Common Acronyms or Terms

ABO
ALL
AML
APTT
BMT
CBC
CLL
CML
DIC
diff
ESR
FFP
Hct
HD
Hgb
IG
ITP
IV
IVIG

CHAPTER OVERVIEW

Chapter 81 reviews the anatomy and physiology of the blood and lymph systems and details common disorders of each system as well as common medical and surgical treatments and diagnostic tests.

✪ Be sure to review the Learning Objectives from the text.

✔ Be sure to FIRST perform Improving Concentration exercises described in the Introduction before proceeding with the next exercise.

Part 1

Using information from the topics outline and key points, answer these statements true (T) or false (F). Correct the false.

1. _____ Blood transfusions are considered a common medical treatment.

2. _____ White blood cell disorders deprive a person of energy and oxygen to carry out the activities of daily living.

3. _____ Hodgkin's disease is considered a hematologic system disorder.

4. _____ Bone marrow transplantation can be used to treat several life-threatening conditions.

5. _____ Platelet disorders can affect a person's ability to fight infections.

Part 2

Using words from the key terms, supply the correct word for the definitions below.

1. _____
   A client's own bone marrow is harvested, frozen, and reinfused.

2. _____
   Sex-linked genetic disorder; lack of factor VIII or IX

3. _____
   White blood cells decrease in number.

4. _____
   Bone marrow received from someone other than client

5. _____
   Malignant hematologic disorder characterized by an abundance of abnormal WBCs

Part 3 Multiple Choice

Circle the letter corresponding to the correct answer.

1. One of the most common hematologic problems that affects people of all ages is:
   a. Hodgkin's disease
   b. Leukopenia
   c. Anemia
   d. Leukemia

2. The two types of acute leukemia are lymphocytic and:
   a. Lymphoblastic
   b. Myelogenous
   c. Thrombocytopenic
   d. Hemophilic

3. The most common cancer in young adults, which is slightly more common in men, is:
   a. Non-Hodgkin's lymphoma
   b. Hodgkin's disease
   c. Acute lymphocytic leukemia (ALL)
   d. Thalassemia

4. The most frequent platelet complication of cancer and its treatments is:
   a. Thrombocytopenia
   b. Leukemia
   c. Leukopenia
   d. Hemophilia

5. Treatment for _____ focuses on the prevention of bleeding episodes:
   a. Thrombocytopenia
   b. Leukemia
   c. Leukopenia
   d. Hemophilia

Part 4 Key Concept

Using information found in one of the key concepts in the chapter, fill in the blanks.

Clients who carry the genetic trait for thalassemia or

_____ _____

disease should be referred for _____

counseling.

82

Cancer

Common Acronyms or Terms

ACS	CHOP	NCI
AFP	CMF	ONS
BCNU	DTIC	Pap test
BMT	EBRT	PIC
BRM	5-FU	PICC
BSE	HCG	PSA
CA	HGFs	TSE
CAF	Ifex	TSPA, TESPA
CCNU	IFN	USDHHS
CEA	ILS	

CHAPTER OVERVIEW

Chapter 82 provides general information regarding the complex group of diseases known as cancer. It discusses diagnostic tests, the nursing process, and common medical and surgical treatments.

✪ Be sure to review the Learning Objectives from the text.

✔ Be sure to FIRST perform Improving Concentration exercises described in the Introduction before proceeding with the next exercise.

Part 1

Using information from the topics outline determine the heading from column I that correlates with the subheading from column II. You may use the information in column II more than once.

Column I

1. _____ Data Collection
2. _____ Prognosis
3. _____ Biotherapy
4. _____ Evaluation
5. _____ Chemotherapy
6. _____ Blood Studies
7. _____ Bone Marrow Transplant
8. _____ Prevention

Column II

a. Common Medical Treatments
b. Common Surgical Treatments
c. Nursing Process
d. Diagnostic Tests
e. General Information

Part 2

Using information contained in the key points complete the statements by filling in the blanks.

1. All persons should learn the _____ warning signs of cancer.

2. Many cancers can be _____ if they are detected _____.

3. The leading cause of cancer death is _____ cancer.

4. Cancer can affect any _____ _____.

5. The _____ major types of cancer are carcinoma, _____, leukemia, and _____.

Part 3

Using the words from the key terms, change one word in the definition to make the statement true.

1. One factor that distinguishes all cancer cells from normal cells is controlled, progressive replication (reproduction).
2. Palliative treatment of tumor-related difficulties is a curative.
3. Neutropenia (increased neutrophils) is a result of cancer treatment.
4. The therapy used to cure metastases is called adjuvant.
5. Malignant neoplasms are usually confined within a capsule and can spread to other tissues.
6. An increase in bone marrow function is known as myelosuppression.
7. If cancer is detected early, while in its tertiary site, prognosis for a cure is favorable.
8. The study of systems, called cytology, can contribute to diagnosis.
9. Carcinogens are substances known to prevent cancer.
10. Sarcomas, including those of bone and muscle, arise in epithelial tissues.

Part 4

Answer these statements true (T) or false (F). Correct the false using information found in the nursing alerts throughout the chapter.

1. _____ The leading cause of cancer deaths in men and women is directly related to cigarette smoking.

2. _____ Radiation, even when correctly managed, is always hazardous to the client.

3. _____ Some clients may perceive radiation as a threat to their energy flow.

4. _____ Cancer survival rates are unaffected by the period of detection.

5. _____ Clients receiving radiation or chemotherapy have an increased risk of infection; therefore, the importance of good handwashing techniques should be stressed.

83

Allergic, Immune, and Autoimmune Disorders

Common Acronyms or Terms

AIDS

HIV

IBD

IDDM

MG

MS

RA

SLE

CHAPTER OVERVIEW

Chapter 83 reviews the anatomy and physiology of the immune system and discusses diagnostic tests as well as hypersensitivity and immune disorders.

✪ Be sure to review the Learning Objectives from the text.

✔ Be sure to FIRST perform Improving Concentration exercises described in the Introduction before proceeding with the next exercise.

Part 1

Using information from the key points, change one word in each statement to make it true.

1. Common manifestations of autoimmune reactions may vary from mild to life-threatening.
2. Allergic disorders occur when the body fails to recognize its own cells.
3. Antibodies are foreign protein substances.
4. Treatment of allergies is directed toward the removal of the allergen and counteracting the antigen response.
5. The major defenders of the immune system are B lymphocytes and T cells.

Part 2

Using information from the nursing alerts in the chapter complete these statements by filling in the blanks.

1. During skin testing and _____ shots, clients are at risk for systemic reactions to _____.

2. Clients should remain in the physician's clinic for _____ minutes following injections for desensitization because of the possibility of _____ reactions.

Part 3

Using information found in the key terms complete the following definitions. The first letter has been supplied for you.

1. A_____: a foreign protein substance

2. I_____: giving of minute doses of allergens subcutaneously

3. A_____: process in which the body begins to produce antibodies against its own healthy cells

4. I_____: antigens that cause an immune response in the body

5. A_____: severe, allergic response

Part 4 Multiple Choice

Circle the letter corresponding to the correct answer.

1. When the skin is covered with tiny blisters that itch and ooze that are usually located in the folds of the neck, elbows, and knees, the condition is called:
   a. Urticaria
   b. Eczema
   c. Hives
   d. Lupus

2. The most frequently mentioned chemical mediator released in the antigen–antibody reaction is:
   a. Epinephrine
   b. Cortisone
   c. Histamine
   d. T cells

3. General treatment of autoimmune diseases is for the most part:
   a. Systemic
   b. Symptomatic
   c. Organ-specific
   d. Immunosuppressive

4. Allergic rhinitis is considered to be in the category of:
   a. Respiratory allergies
   b. Gastrointestinal allergies
   c. Drug allergies
   d. Skin allergies

84

HIV and AIDS

Common Acronyms or Terms

AIDS	INH
ARD	IV
B cells	KS
CDC	PCP
DDC	PCR
DDI	T cells
ELISA	ZDU
HIV	

CHAPTER OVERVIEW

Chapter 84 discusses the human immunodeficiency virus that causes AIDS.

✪ Be sure to review the Learning Objectives from the text.

✔ Be sure to FIRST perform Improving Concentration exercises described in the Introduction before proceeding with the next exercise.

Part 1

Using information from the key points, answer these statements true (T) or false (F). Correct the false.

1. _____ AIDS is always fatal; the emotional, physical, and financial implications are enormous.

2. _____ The terms HIV and AIDS are synonymous.

3. _____ Follow Standard Precautions in caring for all clients to minimize the risk of contracting HIV and other infections.

4. _____ The definition of full-blown AIDS includes a diagnosis based on the T-cell count.

Part 2

Using information from the key terms, complete the following sentences by filling in the blanks.

1. _____ overtakes the biosynthesis of living cells to duplicate itself.

2. _____ _____ _____ is a protozoan infection of the lungs.

3. _____ _____ originate in the bone marrow.

4. HIV has reached _____ proportions, meaning that it affects a particularly wide geographic area.

5. T cells are lymphocytes that mature in the _____.

85

Respiratory Disorders

Common Acronyms or Terms

ABG	flu	PFT
ARDS	INH	Ph
BCg	IPPB	PZA
C & S	IS	RBC
COLD	LS	ROM
COPD	mm Hg	RT
CPAP	MRI	SA
CPT	PaCO$_2$	SOB
CT	PaO$_2$	TB
CWSD	PCP	TCDB
DNS	PD	URI

CHAPTER OVERVIEW

Chapter 85 reviews the anatomy and physiology of the respiratory system and tests, treatments, and common disorders of the respiratory tract.

✪ Be sure to review the Learning Objectives from the text.

✔ Be sure to FIRST perform Improving Concentration exercises described in the Introduction before proceeding with the next exercise.

Part 1

Circle the letter corresponding to the correct answer using information from the topics outline.

1. Pleurisy is considered a:
   a. Chronic Respiratory Disorder
   b. Disorder of the Nose
   c. Common Surgical Treatment
   d. Infectious Respiratory Disorder

2. You are caring for a patient who has had a thoracentesis. You recognize that this is a:
   a. Common Medical Treatment
   b. Common Surgical Treatment
   c. Infectious Respiratory Disorder
   d. Chronic Respiratory Disorder

3. You are researching information on nasal trauma. You realize this subheading can be found under the heading:
   a. Disorders of the Nose
   b. Trauma
   c. Chronic Respiratory Disorders
   d. Neoplasms

4. Laryngitis is considered a(n):
   a. Disorder of the Throat
   b. Chronic Respiratory Disorder
   c. Neoplasm
   d. Infectious Respiratory Disorder

Part 2

Using information from the key points and topics outline complete the sentences by filling in the blanks.

1. When _____ occurs, subsequent changes in the neurologic and cardiovascular systems may develop.

2. Another name for the infectious respiratory disorder known as the common cold is _____ _____.

3. Disorders of the respiratory system may be caused by infections, _____, masses, or _____.

4. Allergic rhinitis, also known as _____ _____, is considered a chronic respiratory disorder.

5. Respiratory disorders may be characterized by _____, changes in respiratory _____, and abnormal _____ sounds.

Part 3

Match the key term in column I with the best definition in column II.

Column I

1. _____ Bronchiectasis
2. _____ Tracheostomy
3. _____ Rhinitis
4. _____ Hemothorax
5. _____ Paracentesis
6. _____ Epistaxis
7. _____ Thoracentesis
8. _____ Pneumothorax
9. _____ Anergic
10. _____ Sinusitis

Column II

a. Puncture of chest wall to remove excess fluid or air

b. Hemorrhage into the lung cavity

c. Inflammation of one or more sinuses located in the head

d. Presence of air in the pleural cavity

e. Cannot appropriately respond to any antigen

f. Puncturing of body cavity for aspiration of fluid

g. Insertion of tube into trachea to allow air flow

h. Chronic dilation of bronchi; walls permanently distended

i. Inflammation of nasal mucous membranes

j. Nosebleed

Part 4

Using information from the nursing alerts in the chapter, answer these statements true (T) or false (F). Correct the false.

1. _____ The client's blood pressure should be taken immediately after a paracentesis or thoracentesis and every 30 minutes until readings are stable.

2. _____ All used facial tissues are contaminated material after collecting sputum specimens.

3. _____ The number of cases of tuberculosis has decreased dramatically over the last several years.

4. _____ Clients with respiratory system disorders should be monitored carefully for signs of respiratory depression when receiving a narcotic.

5. _____ When a client has a chest tube, the water seal must be maintained. If a bottle or connection breaks, this is an emergency. Clamp the chest tubes immediately and summon help.

86

Oxygen Therapy and Respiratory Care

Common Acronyms or Terms

ABG

ARDS

CO_2

COLD

COPD

CPAP

HBO

IPPB

LPM

NC

NRM

O_2

O_2 Sat.

PPV

PRM

PSV

SIMV

SOB

CHAPTER OVERVIEW

Chapter 86 discusses considerations in the provision of oxygen and therapies to assist clients who are having difficulty breathing or are unable to breathe.

✪ Be sure to review the Learning Objectives from the text.

✔ Be sure to FIRST perform Improving Concentration exercises described in the Introduction before proceeding with the next exercise.

Part 1

Using information contained in the topics outline and the key points, complete the sentences by filling in the blanks.

1. Oxygen administration can assist a person to breathe or can be totally _____.

2. The client who is having difficulty breathing may require oxygen with a _____ cannula.

3. Oxygen is _____ to life.

4. The client who is unable to breathe may require a _____.

5. Therapeutic oxygen is like _____.

Part 2

Supply the key term that is described by the definition.

1. Manual resuscitator or Ambu bag: _____ _____ _____.

2. _____ _____ is a high-flow, facial device that provides the most reliable and consistent oxygen enrichment.

3. A respirator, also known as a _____, is a machine that forces air into the lungs.

4. A low-flow device identified by the presence of a bag and the absence of valves is a _____ _____ _____.

5. A _____ _____ measures the amount of oxygen saturation in the blood.

Part 3 Nursing Alert

Using information found throughout the chapter in the nursing alerts, change one word in the following sentences to make them true.

1. _____ The simple mask requires a minimum oxygen flow rate of 10 LPM to prevent carbon dioxide buildup.

2. _____ Do not hypoextend the neck of a person who has experienced a spinal cord injury.

3. _____ The NRM is used only in intensive care units or 2:1 client care situations.

4. _____ Do NOT use a humidifier with a simple mask.

5. _____ The PRM is run at whatever flow rate will keep the bag at least two-thirds inflated.

Part 4 Clinical Thinking

Complete these sentences by filling in the blanks.

1. Mr. Cho is on a ventilator; you realize he must be turned every _____ hours.

2. One of the complications Mr. Cho is at risk for due to the high degree of ventilatory and oxygen support is _____ _____ _____ _____.

87

Digestive Disorders

CHAPTER OVERVIEW

Chapter 87 reviews anatomy and physiology, diagnostic tests, and common treatments and disorders of the digestive system.

✪ Be sure to review the Learning Objectives from the text.

✍ Be sure to FIRST perform Improving Concentration exercises described in the Introduction before proceeding with the next exercise.

Common Acronyms or Terms

ALT	HBV
AN	HCV
AP	HDV
AST	HEV
BAS	I & O
BE	IBD
BRM	IL-2
CA 19-9	IV
CDC	LES
CEA	LFT
CT	LGI
CUC	NPO
DTAD	NSAID
EGD	O & P
ERCP	RBC
ET	TAC
5-FU	TMJ
GA	TNM
GGT	TPN
GI	UGI
H_2	US
HAV	

Part 1

Using the topics outline choose the heading in column I that contains the subheading found in column II. You may use some terms more than once or not at all.

Column I

1. _____ Ileostomy

2. _____ Periodontal Disease

3. _____ Gastric Lavage

4. _____ Endoscopy

5. _____ Total Parenteral Nutrition

Column II

a. Diagnostic Tests

b. Common Medical Treatments

c. Common Surgical Treatments

d. Disorders of the Mouth

e. Disorders of the Liver

Part 2

Use the key points to complete the statement by filling in the blanks.

1. Alcohol is related to _____ and esophageal varices.

2. Ulcers can be found in both the stomach and the _____.

3. Irritable bowel syndrome is usually treated

_____.

4. Diseases of the _____ organs of the GI tract include cholecystitis, cholelithiasis, pancreatitis, and appendicitis.

Part 3 Multiple Choice

Using words and terms from the key terms, circle the letter corresponding to the correct answer.

1. The procedure that allows visualization of the entire colon to the level of the terminal ileum is:
   a. Ileostomy
   b. Gastroscopy
   c. Colonoscopy
   d. Colostomy

2. A mobility disorder of the lower portions of the esophagus in which food cannot pass into the stomach is:
   a. Volvulus
   b. Achalasia
   c. Dyspepsia
   d. Steatorrhea

3. The surgical procedure to remove the entire stomach is a(n):
   a. Gastrectomy
   b. Polypectomy
   c. Achalasia
   d. Ileostomy

4. Telescoping of the bowel is called:
   a. Evisceration
   b. Intussusception
   c. Tenesmus
   d. Cachexia

Part 4 Nursing Alert

Use the information found throughout the chapter in the nursing alerts to answer these statements true (T) or false (F). Correct the false.

1. _____ Aspiration can be fatal.

2. _____ Rectal bleeding and fever are associated symptoms of irritable bowel syndrome.

3. _____ If the nasogastric tube is in the larynx, the client is usually unable to speak.

4. _____ Clients are weaned off steroids quickly and systematically.

5. _____ Lack of fat in the diet causes bile to pool in the gallbladder because it is not needed for fat digestion.

88

Urinary Disorders

Common Acronyms or Terms

AIDS	IPV
ARF	KUB
BPH	PEMG
BUN	RAG
CAPD	RBC
C & S	RP
CGN	SPC (SPUC)
CMG	TURBT
CRF	UA
ECHD	UC
EMG	UPP
ESRD	UTI
ESWL	WBC
HIV	

CHAPTER OVERVIEW

Chapter 88 reviews the anatomy and physiology of the urinary system and discusses treatments and disorders.

✪ Be sure to review the Learning Objectives from the text.

✔ Be sure to FIRST perform Improving Concentration exercises described in the Introduction before proceeding with the next exercise.

Part 1

Using information from the topics outline and the key points, change one word to make the sentence true.

1. Hydronephrosis is an infectious disorder.

2. Most incontinence is curable.

3. Dialysis is a common medical treatment.

4. Disorders of the kidneys affect most body systems.

5. Benign renal cysts would be located under the heading of trauma.

Part 2

Complete the definition using words from the key terms. The number of letters in each word is indicated in parentheses.

1. _____(10) allows visualization of the inside of the bladder.

2. _____(8) are bladder muscles that push the urine out.

3. _____ (8) is inflammation of the urinary bladder.

4. _____(9) is a physician who treats diseases of the urinary system.

5. _____(8) assumes the work of a damaged, nonfunctioning kidney.

Part 3 Key Concepts

Choose the best answer based on your review of key concepts presented throughout the chapter.

1. Urodynamic tests are the tests of choice in many cases because:
   a. They are usually done in an operating room.
   b. They are the treatment of choice for stress incontinence.
   c. They provide the best information about kidney function.
   d. They are safer than x-ray procedures that require an IV dye.

2. Evaluation of renal function requires:
   a. Hemodialysis
   b. Urodynamic testing
   c. Strictly timed urine and blood collection
   d. Surgical intervention

3. Neoplasms may present problems in renal function by:
   a. Interfering with bladder training
   b. Obstructing urinary flow
   c. Causing nephrotoxicity
   d. Interfering with lithotripsy

4. In this form of dialysis the semipermeable membrane is the person's own peritoneum:
   a. Hemodialysis
   b. Peritoneal dialysis
   c. Hemofiltration
   d. Hemodiafiltration

89

Male Reproductive Disorders

Common Acronyms or Terms

ABP

ARRP

BPH

CBP

NBP

PSA

TSE

TURP

UA/UC

CHAPTER OVERVIEW

Chapter 89 reviews the anatomy and physiology, common medical and surgical treatments, and various disorders of the male reproductive system.

✪ Be sure to review the Learning Objectives from the text.

✔ Be sure to FIRST perform Improving Concentration exercises described in the Introduction before proceeding with the next exercise.

Part 1

Complete the sentence using information from the topics outline and the key points.

1. Priapism is an _____ disorder.

2. Most _____ cancers occur between the ages of 18 and 35.

3. Hydrocele is a kind of _____ disorder.

4. _____ of the spermatic cord is an emergency.

5. All men over the age of _____ years should have a rectal digital examination.

Part 2

Using information from the key terms, change one word to make the sentence true.

1. Hypospadias is the term for testicles that have not descended to their normal place.
2. Phimosis refers to abnormal and persistent penile erection without sexual stimulation.
3. Epididymitis is inflammation of the testes.
4. A varicocele is a type of testicular tumor that often remains localized until late in the disease course.
5. Orchitis is accumulation of fluid in the space between the membrane covering the testicle and the testicle itself.

Part 3

Answer these statements true (T) or false (F). Correct the false.

1. _____ The prostate-specific antigen (PSA) test detects a glucocorticoid found only in the tissue of the prostate gland.

2. _____ Sitz baths are usually ordered after a perineal prostatectomy.

3. _____ Mumps before puberty may cause orchitis, resulting in sterility.

4. _____ When the urethral meatus is located on the underside of the penis, the condition is called hypospadias.

5. _____ Circumcision at an early age prevents cancer of the penis.

6. _____ Clients who have had a radical prostatectomy have a urethral catheter in place for about 2 days.

7. _____ Including skin cancer, cancer of the prostate is the most common cancer in men.

8. _____ Benign prostatic hyperplasia (BPH) is a common condition in which the prostate gland enlarges.

9. _____ Except for leukemia and lymphoma, penile cancer is the most common form of cancer in men between the ages of 20 and 34.

10. _____ Orchiopexy involves suturing the testes to the scrotal sac to fixate them.

90

Female Reproductive Disorders

Common Acronyms or Terms

AC

ACS

AP

BSE

CA

CMF

D & C

DES

DVT

GYN

HPV

HRT

in situ

IUD

PAP

PID

PMS

STD

TSS

US

CHAPTER OVERVIEW

Chapter 90 reviews the anatomy and physiology, diagnostic tests, common medical and surgical treatments, and various disorders of the female reproductive system.

✪ Be sure to review the Learning Objectives from the text.

✔ Be sure to FIRST perform Improving Concentration exercises described in the Introduction before proceeding with the next exercise.

Part 1

Using headings and subheadings from the topic outline, determine the proper heading in column II to accompany the subheading in column I. You may use the headings more than once.

Column I

1. _____ Vulvodynia
2. _____ Prolapsed Uterus
3. _____ Pelvic Exenteration
4. _____ Cystocele
5. _____ Pelvic Examination
6. _____ Metrorrhagia
7. _____ Endometriosis
8. _____ Dilation and Curettage
9. _____ Dysmenorrhea
10. _____ Breast Examination

Column II

a. Common Surgical Treatments

b. Diagnostic Tests

c. Disorders Related to the Menstrual Cycle

d. Inflammatory Disorders

e. Structural Disorders

Part 2

Supply the word from the key terms that corresponds with the definition.

1. _____ is bleeding between menstrual periods.

2. _____ is downward displacement of the bladder toward the vaginal orifice.

3. _____ is a plastic surgery revision of the breast.

4. _____ is inflammation of the cervix.

5. _____ provides direct visualization of the uterus and accessory organs.

Part 3 Nursing Alert

Use the information found in the nursing alerts throughout the chapter to answer these statements true (T) or false (F). Correct the false.

1. _____ Pap smears should be done between a woman's menstrual periods.

2. _____ Toxic shock syndrome or another serious infection may occur if a woman forgets or cannot remove a tampon.

3. _____ Women who are anorexic often experience menorrhagia.

4. _____ A woman who has had PID is no more likely to have an ectopic pregnancy than a woman with normal health.

5. _____ Postmenopausal bleeding is often caused by a myoma.

Part 4 Clinical Teaching

Use information found in the key concepts in the chapter to fill in the blanks below.

1. You are informing Ms. Markelson of the importance of breast self-examination. You recall from your reading that about _____% of all breast cancers are discovered by self-examination.

2. You are also aware that a woman who has had a mastectomy should check her _____ _____ and scar area because these are common sites for _____.

91

Gerontology: The Aging Adult

Common Acronyms or Terms

ALF

LTC

TPN

VA

CHAPTER OVERVIEW

Chapter 91 presents an overview of the aging adult and related special care needs. The role of the nurse in providing care to the aging adult in a variety of settings is discussed.

✪ Be sure to review the Learning Objectives from the text.

✍ Be sure to FIRST perform Improving Concentration exercises described in the Introduction before proceeding with the next exercise.

Part 1

Match the following subheadings in column I with the major headings in column II.

Column I

1. _____ Substance Abuse

2. _____ Senior Day Care

3. _____ Communication

4. _____ Personal Hygiene Needs

5. _____ Safety

Column II

a. Elder Abuse

b. Special Concerns of the Aging Adult

c. Helping the Older Adult Meet Emotional Needs

d. Helping the Older Adult Meet Basic Needs

e. Care Settings for Older Adults

Part 2 Key Term Definitions

Fill in the term or terms for the definition provided.

1. _____
   Choking

2. _____
   Exhaustion and frustration of daily obligations related to care of an older person

3. _____
   Without teeth

4. _____
   Easily broken

5. _____
   A sensorineural hearing problem that first affects the ability to hear high-frequency sounds (eg, F, PH, S, and SH sounds).

6. _____
   Temporary relief and rest for adult children of seniors

Part 3 Multiple Choice

Circle the letter corresponding to the correct answer.

1. Which of the following phrases might an aging client with presbycusis have difficulty hearing?
   a. Shake the solution first, then evenly pour it into two equal doses.
   b. Mix the medication with water in a cup and drink it all.
   c. Don't add milk to the drug and don't drink milk until an hour after taking it.
   d. Never mix the two antibiotics unless the doctor tells you to.

2. Which of the following would be an appropriate action for a client with Sjögren's syndrome?
   a. Instructing the client to rub eyes during the day to stimulate secretion of moisture
   b. Suggesting the client wear glasses to decrease drying of eyes
   c. Asking the doctor to provide a prescription for artificial tears
   d. Limiting the client's fluid intake and intake of foods high in salt

3. Clients with presbyopia:
   a. May notice difficulty reading with bright light in the room
   b. Read better with bifocals to allow for far and near vision
   c. Need an antibiotic to cure the infection in each eye
   d. May need speech therapy to resolve communication problems

Part 4

Complete the following fill-in-the-blank or short answer exercises.

1. A _____ _____ is any adult who is put in jeopardy of being abused or neglected.

2. _____ _____ comprises emotional, physical, and sexual abuse, financial exploitation, or neglect of older persons.

3. List two factors for determining the choice of residence for an aging adult. _____

4. Name four care settings for older adults.
   _____ _____
   _____ _____

5. Discuss measures for emotional and psychological support of older adults. _____
   _____
   _____
   _____ _____
   _____
   _____
   _____

92

Dementias and Related Disorders

Common Acronyms or Terms

AD	BPRS	IADL	RPR
ADL	CT	ID	SDAT
ADRDA	EEG	MID	SPECT
AIDS	FADL	MRI	VDRL
ALT	HD	PET	

CHAPTER OVERVIEW

Chapter 92 discusses forms of dementia, confusion, and delirium and their impact on the older person. Nursing implications associated with these conditions is addressed.

✪ Be sure to review the Learning Objectives from the text.

✔ Be sure to FIRST perform Improving Concentration exercises described in the Introduction before proceeding with the next exercise.

Part 1

Complete these sentences by filling in the blanks.

1. If looking for information related to Confusion, Delirium, and Dementia you would look under the _____ major heading in the chapter.

2. The second major heading in the chapter covers _____ of _____.

3. Treatment for Alzheimer's disease is _____; there is no known cure.

4. _____ care and support services are necessary for caregivers of clients with dementia.

Part 2

Match the term(s) in column I with the definition in column II.

Column I

1. _____ Apraxia
2. _____ Dementia
3. _____ Ambiguous loss
4. _____ Catastrophic reaction
5. _____ Pseudodementia
6. _____ Confabulation
7. _____ Delirium
8. _____ Confusion

Column II

a. The debilitating confusion (of the family) about whether their living loved one is still with them or is gone

b. Problems carrying out purposeful movements

c. Term used to describe a condition in which a client has the appearance of dementia but whose confusion results from depression

d. Becoming agitated when confronted with situations that are too overwhelming or difficult

e. Fabricating details of events

f. Impairment of mental function, means poor judgment, impaired memory, and disorientation to time, place, situation, or person

g. Confusion, sleep disturbances, and restlessness progressing to anxiety, delusions, hallucination, or fear

h. Literally means "mind away"; chronic, irreversible condition that affects cognitive function, eventually interfering with a person's ability to function normally and provide self-care

Part 3

Indicate if the following actions are appropriate (A) or inappropriate (I).

1. _____ Including information such as the client's flu shots and Pneumovax immunizations in the nursing history and physical

2. _____ Determining if an AD client's sleep problems are disruptive for family members

3. _____ Being firm and strong with AD clients who are physically aggressive and restraining these clients to help them see that they cannot overpower others

4. _____ Reasoning with an AD client who is paranoid and delusional and believes people on television are in the room by explaining that television is not real

5. _____ Monitoring an AD client closely for suicide, particularly in the early stages of AD

6. _____ Recognizing a history of falls or unsteady gait as danger signs of problems with walking without assistance

7. _____ Providing AD clients with daily baths in the morning with high levels of water to soak the body totally because body odor is distressing for the client with AD

8. _____ Maintaining hydration in the client with AD by providing fluids as requested to meet the more acute sense of thirst that older people experience

Part 4

Complete the following short answer or fill-in-the-blank exercises.

1. Name three theories of causes of Alzheimer's disease (AD). _____
_____
_____

2. _____-_____
and _____-_____
memory impairment are symptoms in identification of dementia.

3. Name two of the three major physiologic changes that occur in the brain of a person with AD. _____
_____

4. Multi-infarct dementia can be distinguished from AD in the following ways: it has a _____ onset; it progresses in a _____ fashion (not gradually), and it may coexist with other _____.

5. _____ dementias are related to drug overdoses; _____ dementias can occur after untreated end-stage renal disease or hepatic failure.

6. Pain control is important because clients with dementia may experience pain but may be unable to _____ it.

93

Psychiatric Nursing

Common Acronyms or Terms

ADL

AH

AIDS

AP

APA

BPD

BPRS

CIC

CNS

CT

DCH

DISCUS

DSM-IV

ECG

ECT

EEG

EP

EPSE

ETOH

GP/SP

HHA

HI

KELS

LOC

MAO

MAOI

MI/CD

MI & D

MMPI

MMSE

MRI

NMS

NSAID

OCD

OT

PADS

PCA

PET

PD

PTSD

REBT

REM

SA

SI

SIB

SPECT

SSDI

SSRI

SX

SZ

TAT

TCD

TD

T-Hold

TR

VH

WBC

W/D

WHO

CHAPTER OVERVIEW

Chapter 93 discusses the care of clients with alterations in mental health. An overview of mental health, mental illness, and types of psychiatric therapy in the inpatient settings is presented. Mental health nursing skills are addressed.

✪ Be sure to review the Learning Objectives from the text.

✤ Be sure to FIRST perform Improving Concentration exercises described in the Introduction before proceeding with the next exercise.

Part 1

Complete the statements by filling in the blanks.

1. The major heading in which treatment centers and resources are found in this chapter is _____.

2. Information related to electroconvulsive therapy is found under the major heading _____.

3. Today most mentally ill people are treated in the _____.

4. One of the most common mood disorders is _____, which is a major cause of suicide.

5. Many psychiatric clients who use their medication are able to live _____ in the community.

Part 2

Supply the term for the definition provided.

1. _____
   Outward manifestation of subjective emotions

2. _____
   Inability to sit still; agitation, tapping, rocking, pacing, and marching in place

3. _____
   Depressed mood most of the day or markedly diminished or loss of interest or pleasure in all, or most, activities

4. _____
   Fear of impending danger

5. _____
   Involuntary writhing movements of fingers, toes, and extremities and back and sideways head jerks, usually to one side

6. _____
   Stupor, muscle rigidity

7. _____
   Repetitive behavior (eg, handwashing, cleaning) or mental acts (eg, counting, constant praying) that the person feels driven to perform, sometimes constantly

8. _____
   Reaction to stress

9. _____
   Has commonly come to mean mental illness, combined with chemical dependency (MI/CD)

10. _____
    Involuntary, coordinated rhythmic movements, jerking, tremors, twisting, tongue movements

Part 3

Correct the following definitions by moving the words to the correct definition in this part.

1. *Neuroleptic malignant syndrome (NMS)* is difficulty in speaking.
2. *Psychotropic* means occurring when no specific causative agent is located.
3. *Dystonia* is a therapeutic environment in which all aspects of the surroundings (physical and social) are designed to promote health and to enable clients to cope with life's demands.
4. A *functional disorder* is noisy (with words, singing, or just sounds), or not speaking.
5. *Milieu therapy* is an antipsychotic (major tranquilizer), effective in treating "positive" symptoms of psychosis: hallucinations, delusions, paranoia, severe agitation, hyperactivity, combativeness, and feelings of unreality.
6. In *mutism* conversation does not make sense, dwelling on one subject, or returning to the same subject.
7. *Oculogyric crisis* is a rare, life-threatening complication of neuroleptic medications.
8. *Schizophrenia* is backward rolling of eyes, non-movement side effects, including dry mouth, blurred vision, constipation, thick tongue, weight gain, sleepiness, tachycardia.
9. *Neuroleptic drugs* (mood modifiers) include antipsychotics, antianxiety/sedative–hypnotics, mood stabilizers, and antidepressants.
10. *Perseverate* is a group of psychotic disorders that have two or more of the following positive symptoms: delusions, hallucinations, disorganized speech, grossly disorganized behavior, and catatonia.

Part 4

Complete these short answer exercises by filling in the blanks.

1. At least 50% of all suicides can be attributed to a _____ disorder.

2. Diagnosis of a major depressive episode includes five or more symptoms and at least one symptom must be _____.

3. The mood disorder in which broad mood variations range from mania to major depression is _____ (BPD).

4. Give an example of a personality disorder, anxiety disorder, and psychosis. _____

5. A client who is admitted to a mental health facility placed by the police is under a _____ hold.

6. Many mental health and geriatric units use _____ technique or reality orientation.

7. _____ therapy involves having a client interact with a kitten or puppy.

8. Psychotropic drugs such as antipsychotic or neuroleptic drugs may have side effects such as parkinsonism or general dyskinesia. These adverse effects are called _____ side effects.

9. The rights of the client are protected through _____ rights legislation, _____ adult legislation, and _____.

10. The program of nursing care for the very mentally ill client involves _____ care, _____ skills, and building _____ skills.

Part 5

Match the nursing action in column I with the client in column II for whom it would be most appropriate.

Column I

1. _____ Know whereabouts and condition of each resident at all times; 15-minute checks are a minimum.

2. _____ Maintaining a quiet atmosphere is important.

3. _____ Care includes physical protection; allow active people a wide scope of activity for their surplus energy.

4. _____ Recognize the person's feelings without judgment; defensiveness is ineffective and dangerous.

5. _____ Be firm but kind, avoid familiarity and arguments, keep such persons from irritating others, and try to keep them occupied.

Column II

a. Overactive person

b. Hypomanic or manic person

c. Hostile or combative person

d. Suicidal person

e. Highly disturbed person

94

Substance Abuse

Common Acronyms or Terms

AA

ACOA

APA

CD

CNS

COA

$D_5W/2NS$

DTs

EEG

ETOH

FAS

LSD

$MgSO_4$

MI/CD

MJ

NA

NSAID

OTC

PCP

RET

THC

W/D

CHAPTER OVERVIEW

Chapter 94 discusses the abuse of harmful mood-altering chemicals and resulting care needs. The role of the nurse in caring for those with addictions is addressed.

✪ Be sure to review the Learning Objectives from the text.

✤ Be sure to FIRST perform Improving Concentration exercises described in the Introduction before proceeding with the next exercise.

Part 1

Complete the following exercises related to titles of the major headings (subheadings provide a hint) and key points in the chapter.

1. S_____ A_____
   and C_____ D_____
   (causes, nature, management)

2. D_____ and R_____
   (immediate treatment, long-term follow-up and treatment)

3. Major precipitating factors of chemical abuse include _____ and low ____
   _____.

4. The _____ or enabler is a key figure in alcoholism.

5. Nurses are _____ likely to abuse substances than the general population.

Part 2

Supply the key term defined below.

1. _____ _____
   Drugs, some without pharmacologic effects of their own, are used as adjunctive therapy.

2. _____ _____
   Delusions and vivid and terrifying auditory, visual, and tactile hallucinations, (eg, bugs crawling on the skin), which may last from a few days to several weeks

3. _____ _____
Adverse conditioning in the chronic alcoholic who is unable to maintain sobriety

4. _____
Periods of total amnesia, often occur with excessive use

5. _____ _____ (CD)
Any drug that is abused, including alcohol, marijuana, or drugs prescribed by a physician that are used in a maladaptive pattern of substance use leading to clinically significant impairment or distress

6. _____ _____ (DTs)
Delusions and hallucinations occurring during alcohol withdrawal; an indicator of a severe toxic state in stage 3 withdrawal

7. _____
Process of removing a drug and its physiologic effects from the addicted person's body

8. _____ _____
Is life-threatening and can occur when a starving person receives carbohydrates too quickly

9. _____ _____
Maladaptive pattern of substance use leading to clinically significant impairment or distress

10. _____
Characteristic symptoms occurring when use of drugs is stopped or taking the same or related substances to avoid symptoms

Part 3

Complete the following statements or short answer exercises.

1. Any drug can be abused, including _____, marijuana, or drugs _____ by a physician.

2. _____ is needing more of a drug to cause intoxication or experiencing decreased effects from previously sufficient amounts.

3. _____ is considered one of the most addicting drugs available; stimulates constriction of blood vessels.

4. Athletes showing symptoms such as irritability, edema, insomnia, or electrolyte imbalance should be questioned about the use of _____ _____.

5. Coffee, tea, chocolate, and soft drinks all contain _____, and dependence on it is a physical reality.

6. Theories related to the causes of chemical dependency (CD) include _____ factors theory, _____ theory, _____ and _____ theories, and dual disorder, which involves _____ illness combined with chemical dependency.

7. The three most important defense mechanisms in substance abuse are _____, _____, and _____.

8. In an emergency department admission of a person intoxicated with some unknown substance, the nurse should anticipate _____ behaviors.

9. Routinely used supplements administered to chemically dependent clients include _____, _____ _____, and a multivitamin with iron.

10. The goals of treatment during detoxification and recovery are to assist clients to address _____ problems associated with abuse and to understand the _____ of dependence.

Part 4

Circle the letter corresponding to the correct answer.

1. Roy Roders is admitted after a motorcycle accident. You discover in your nursing assessment that he has abused cocaine for the past year. You would build into his plan of care the need to:
   a. Monitor his pulse for a decreased rate because depressant effect of cocaine withdrawal.
   b. Maintain a steady noise in the environment with radio or TV to prevent depression during withdrawal.
   c. Encourage the client to walk around the hospital unit to promote socialization with other clients and prevent isolation.
   d. Monitor his respirations and prepare to give res-

piratory stimulants to counteract respiratory depression.

2. Mrs. Jachil is admitted for detoxification from barbiturate abuse. Her husband inquires about drug abuse and the use of programs. You would be accurate if you informed him that:

   a. The 12-step program has been effective in curing persons who abuse drugs.

   b. Physical abuse cannot occur unless psychological dependence is present so both must be treated.

   c. Treating the substance abuser alone is not enough; the family also needs intensive counseling.

   d. Getting Mrs. Jachil to reduce her abuse of barbiturates is a sign she will soon become drug free.

3. Mr. Palmer is scheduled to receive Antabuse therapy. You would hold the drug and notify the physician if you discovered which of the following during your nursing assessment?

   a. He had his last drink of alcohol about 36 hours ago.

   b. He had a recent experience of left-sided weakness.

   c. His wife is pregnant and in her second trimester.

   d. He has a strong family history of alcohol abuse.

95

Extended Care and Rehabilitation

Common Acronyms or Terms

ADL	ICF
ALS	ICU
B & C	MI
CF	MVA
CHT	PM & R
CPM	PROM
CVA	ROM
ECF	SNF
FADL	TBI
FES	TENS
HD	UAP
IADL	

CHAPTER OVERVIEW

Chapter 95 discusses lifestyle and housing alternatives available to clients outside the hospital. Nursing care provided to clients in these settings is addressed.

✪ Be sure to review the Learning Objectives from the text.

✔ Be sure to FIRST perform Improving Concentration exercises described in the Introduction before proceeding with the next exercise.

PART 1

Complete the following statements by filling in the blanks.

1. The major heading Extended Care includes sub-headings on subacute care or transitional facilities, _____ care facilities, and _____ _____ options.

2. Clients may move from one type of _____ _____ to another, as their needs change.

3. The least _____ type of care should be given to promote the client's independent functioning.

4. The major heading _____ _____ has subheadings addressing the rehabilitation team and the community resources.

5. _____ assists in strengthening exercises to prevent falls or other injury and to provide mobility.

Part 2

Supply the correct term for the definition provided.

1. _____ _____
   One way to facilitate independent living; programs give older adults the opportunity to age in place, while maintaining their independence, individuality, privacy, and dignity.

2. _____ _____
   A special high-rise or other building designated for a specific group. These buildings may contain free-standing apartments, with no supervision or with minimal supervision. A person must qualify to live there and usually receives subsidized rent on a sliding scale, based on income.

3. _____ _____
   _____ _____ (TENS)
   Electrical therapy that assists in pain management

4. _____ _____ _____ (ICFs)
   Provide fewer services and less extensive care than SNFs. They provide room, board, and nursing care. A licensed nurse is usually not required to be on duty 24 hours a day.

5. _____

Young people who are physically or mentally challenged attending regular classes in school, participating in school activities, and having the opportunity to mingle with others their own age

6. _____

Bladder or bowel lacking nerve stimulation

7. _____

Medical specialty involved in the fabrication of braces and splints

8. _____

Physician who specializes in rehabilitation, sometimes called physical medicine and rehabilitation (PM & R) specialists

9. _____

The fabrication and adjustment of prostheses (artificial limbs)

10. _____ _____ _____ (SNF)

Provides 24-hour care and must have a licensed nurse on duty. This facility provides rehabilitation services, special diets, and access to pharmacy and laboratory services.

Part 3

Identify the following actions as appropriate (A) or inappropriate (I).

1. _____ Referring the client who is physically challenged due to an injury with no possibility of complete recovery for rehabilitation

2. _____ Expecting the client who is adjusting to a physical or mental challenge to undergo shock, denial, anger, bargaining, depression, then acceptance reactions

3. _____ Encouraging the client in rehabilitation to relax and become dependent on staff for a short time to rest and recuperate

4. _____ Suggesting clients get electrical outlets installed higher off the floor to promote easy reach

5. _____ Instructing clients who are wheelchair bound to take tub baths instead of showers

6. _____ Suggesting the hemiplegic client place clothing on the unaffected arm or leg first and to undress the affected arm or leg first

Part 4

Complete the following exercises by filling in the blanks.

1. Clients whose sensation or mobility is impaired are at high risk for _____

_____.

2. To assist a client to establish regular patterns of voiding, assist them to void every _____ hours and gradually increase the interval.

3. A client who is _____ is paralyzed on one side of the body; in the client who is _____ all four extremities and possibly the trunk are paralyzed.

4. Chronic conditions such as arthritis and low back pain often require ongoing nonpharmacologic pain management, as well as _____ and _____ exercises.

5. _____ ADL include aspects of self-care such as dressing, bathing, toileting and continence, whereas _____ ADL involve more complex living skills such as food preparation, laundry, and money management.

96

Ambulatory and Home Care Nursing

Common Acronyms or Terms

ACS	FHC	NPO
CHC	HCA	PCA
CHHA	HHA	PCP
ECG	HMO	PHN
EHS	IV	
EMT	NAHC	

CHAPTER OVERVIEW

Chapter 96 discusses the varied settings in which health care services are provided outside the inpatient setting. Nursing care provided to clients during same-day surgery and in home and community settings is addressed.

✪ Be sure to review the Learning Objectives from the text.

✔ Be sure to FIRST perform Improving Concentration exercises described in the Introduction before proceeding with the next exercise.

Part 1

Indicate if the following statements are true (T) or false (F) based on your review of the major headings and key points.

1. _____ Information about private clinics and health centers can be found under the major heading Ambulatory Healthcare Sites.

2. _____ The major heading Home Care contains information about the family/community health center.

3. _____ Home care nursing is the fastest growing segment of the healthcare delivery system.

4. _____ Home care nurses must follow the scheduled hours set for them by clients and the physician.

5. _____ The home health agency ultimately has the primary responsibility for the personal safety of the home health nurse.

Part 2

Supply the term that is defined below.

1. _____
   Defibrillation

2. _____
   Plan that outlines protocols for the management of a specific disorder that is considered ambulatory care sensitive (ACS)

3. _____
   Coexisting disorders

4. _____
   Plan that outlines protocols for the management of a specific disorder.

5. _____
   Entry points used to perform complex abdominal and chest surgery

6. _____
   Clients with noncritical conditions

Part 3

Using the word list below, correct the following statements by changing the incorrect term.

1. The nurse in an ambulatory healthcare site will *perform* sterile procedures, including minor surgery.
2. The nurse will also *write* prescriptions to pharmacies.
3. The nurse will *increase* the client's blood sugar level when working in specialized clinics.
4. In family/community health centers nurse practitioners often provide *secondary* healthcare to people of all ages.
5. Nurses in the emergency department or emergicenter often *perform surgery* in the event of multiple admissions at one time to determine which clients require immediate attention.

Primary

Triage

Measure

Call in

Assist with

Part 4

Indicate if the following activities would be appropriate (A) or inappropriate (I).

1. _____ The nurse performing special nonnursing procedures, such as laboratory procedures or electrocardiograms when working in an ambulatory healthcare site

2. _____ Encouraging clients with underlying disorders to complete paperwork and laboratory tests so they will be prepared for day surgery instead of inpatient surgery

3. _____ Giving instructions to clients verbally by telephone and in writing and at the last preoperative office visit when the client is scheduled for day surgery

4. _____ Performing specific preparations, such as preoperative scrub and shaving or drawing of blood the day before the procedure

5. _____ Instructing the client to drive in early and park close to the building so there is less walking needed before driving home after the procedure

Part 5

Complete the following statements by filling in the blanks.

1. Several types of agencies provide home care services; they include _____ agencies, nursing _____, _____ companies, and _____ programs.

2. State two locations in which hospice care may be delivered. _____ _____

3. Older adults or people with chronic, disabling conditions may require _____ care.

4. List standard duties the LPN/LVN might perform in home care. _____ _____ _____ _____ _____

5. State five employee safety guidelines for the home health nurse. _____ _____ _____ _____ _____

97

Hospice Nursing

Common Acronyms or Terms

ABHR	DNR	PCA
AIDS	IV	TENS
DNH	MOM	WHO
DNI	NHO	

CHAPTER OVERVIEW

Chapter 97 discusses the use of hospice care for terminally ill persons. The role of the nurse in hospice care is addressed.

✪ Be sure to review the Learning Objectives from the text.

✔ Be sure to FIRST perform Improving Concentration exercises described in the Introduction before proceeding with the next exercise.

Part 1

Complete the following fill-in-the blank exercises related to the major headings or key points.

1. The first major heading in the chapter is
   E_____ of the _____
   _____

2. Information in the chapter related to the goals and characteristics of a hospice can be found under the major heading The H_____
   C_____.

3. Information in this chapter related to pain management and what to do when a client dies is located under the major heading R_____ of the
   _____ Nurse.

4. _____ care may be necessary for family members (of terminally ill clients).

5. The goal of pain and symptom management is
   _____ without unwanted
   _____ _____

Part 2

Supply the correct term for the definition provided.

1. _____
   Neurosurgery performed to sever (cut) the pain pathway

2. _____
   Assisting medications added to potentiate (enhance) an opioid's effects or to treat other symptoms

3. _____
   Grieving; part of the process of dealing with a loved one's death

4. _____
   Palliative surgery done in any body part to relieve pressure or obstruction by removing part of a tumor

5. _____
   Care of terminally ill persons, treating them with dignity

6. _____
   Symptom control

7. _____
   Designated significant others

8. _____
   Taking a break

9. _____
   Very difficult or impossible to arouse

10. _____
    Gradually increase of the dose of a narcotic

Part 3

Answer these statements true (T) or false (F).

1. _____ The client with anorexia needs good mouth care and frequent small meals.

2. _____ Nauseated clients should lie on their left sides and receive antiemetics.

3. _____ The client with diarrhea can be assisted by a high-residue diet, which decreases stimulation.

4. _____ The client with respiratory distress may obtain relief from a fan to cool the room and elevating the head of the bed.

5. _____ Before treating constipation it should be determined whether a bowel obstruction exists.

6. _____ Clients with insomnia need stimulating music before bedtime to promote exhaustion.

7. _____ Clients in pain receive relief most often through intramuscular medication.

8. _____ Terminal clients should be encouraged to maintain physical activity and exercise for as long as possible.

9. _____ A major adverse side effect of opiates is sedation, sometimes with respiratory depression.

10. _____ Staff members must consider dying children in terms of their developmental levels and levels of understanding.

Part 4

Complete the following by filling in the blanks.

1. Hospice care focuses on four areas of human needs, which include _____, _____/_____, _____/_____, and _____ needs.

2. The goal of hospice is symptom control, which aims to _____ symptoms that interfere with the client's _____ of life, without causing unnecessary and _____ side effects.

3. State three sample criteria for admission to a hospice. _____

4. The two greatest fears terminally ill clients in hospice have are that they will be _____ _____ to die and the fear of _____.

5. Hospice nurses _____ the client's ongoing condition and _____ findings with team members.

98

Leadership and Management

Common Acronyms or Terms

CLTC

D/C

ECF

MAR

NFLPN

NLN

SNF

TO

UAP

VO

WWW

CHAPTER OVERVIEW

Chapter 98 discusses the role of nurses as leaders in various healthcare settings. The scope of leadership responsibilities of the LPN/LVN is addressed.

✪ Be sure to review the Learning Objectives from the text.

✔ Be sure to first perform Improving Concentration exercises described in the Introduction before proceeding with the next exercise.

Part 1

Match the subjects in column I with the major headings under which they can be found in column II.

Column I

1. _____ Leadership styles

2. _____ Team leader or charge nurse

3. _____ Operative orders

4. _____ Telephone or verbal orders

5. _____ The Internet

Column II

a. Continuity of Nursing Care

b. Advanced Certification in Long-Term Care

c. Technology in Healthcare

d. Transcribing or Checking Physicians' Orders

e. Specific Management Skills

f. The Nursing Team

Part 2

Fill in the blanks to complete the following statements related to the key points.

1. The role of all nurses, including LPNs, is _____.

2. Several different leadership styles exist. There is no _____ or _____ style; any of them can be _____.

3. A wide variety of specialty certifications are in place for nurses. LPNs, for example, can be _____ certified in long-term care.

Part 3

Supply the term that matches the definition provided.

1. _____ leadership
   Is self-directed with little or no input from staff

2. _____ leadership
   Is policy-minded, with leaders relying on established protocols for decision-making

3. _____ _____
   Additional education

4. _____ leadership
   Is people oriented and tries to guide staff in the right direction

5. _____
   Leadership style with the least structure, with loosely structured goals with no firm guidelines

6. _____
   Involves sorting calls to decide which are life-threatening situations and should be referred to 911 or other emergency services

Part 4

Complete the following by filling in the blanks.

1. According to the National League for Nursing (NLN) "LPNs/LVNs are concerned with basic

   _____ _____

   and _____ care for people of

   all ages. . . ."

2. State five entry-level skills or competencies the LPN/LVN needs to demonstrate. _____

   _____

   _____

   _____

3. The LPN/LVN who acts as a charge nurse is responsible for getting _____ report,

   _____ clients to staff members, determining client _____,

   and handling _____.

4. To assign duties to other members of the nursing team, the charge nurse must know the client, so the first thing the charge nurse will do is _____

   _____.

5. When transcribing medication orders the charge nurse should read _____ orders and always do _____ orders first.

6. The charge nurse should make sure that the nursing student or other unlicensed person never takes

_____ or _____

orders.

Part 5

Indicate if the following actions would be appropriate (A) or inappropriate (I).

1. _____ Using a computer to assist in developing a nursing care plan

2. _____ Leaving clients alone at night and keeping lights out in the room, particularly if the client has dementia or paranoia

3. _____ Reducing the amount of pain medication given to clients at night because pain usually decreases

4. _____ Providing clients who are NPO with a snack with 1 AM medications because food will help the client rest after being aroused

5. _____ Providing medications such as laxatives and vaginal suppositories to a client in the evening

99

Career Opportunities and Job-Seeking

Common Acronyms or Terms

CAT

CEU

ECF

NAPNES

NCLEX

NFLPN

OSHA

CHAPTER OVERVIEW

Chapter 99 discusses career planning for the graduate nurse. Licensure and employment concerns are addressed.

✪ Be sure to review the Learning Objectives from the text.

✍ Be sure to FIRST perform Improving Concentration exercises described in the Introduction before proceeding with the next exercise.

Part 1

Fill in the blanks to complete the following statements related to major headings and key points.

1. Information related to policies can be located under the major heading _____.

2. To explore information about setting up a personal nursing file, the student would look under the major heading _____ _____.

3. You can conduct a job _____, _____ for a position, and take _____ _____ courses via the Internet.

4. Your nursing education is just _____. You will be _____ the rest of your professional life.

5. Nurses should become involved in professional _____ and in their local _____.

Part 2

Supply the correct term to match the definition provided.

1. _____
   Graduation or a beginning

2. _____
   Moving or transferring licensure to another state

3. _____
   Period of internship before being considered full-fledged LPNs or RNs or benefit-earning members of the staff

4. _____
   Licensure without examination

5. _____
   Medical pool that recruits nurses to work in facilities that need extra help for special duty clients, during busy periods, or for vacation coverage

6. _____
   There are two types; one type emphasizes strengths and abilities, and the other lists experience chronologically.

7. _____
   A growing area of nursing employment. It provides healthcare facilities with a cost-effective way to manage clients. Nurses require specialized in-service education before they can perform telehealth services.

Part 3

Complete the following statements by filling in the blanks.

1. Your first task on graduation from an approved nursing program is to make arrangements to take the _____ licensing examination to practice.

2. The LPN's role _____ in each state and in every facility.

3. List five places the graduate nurse may find general employment opportunities; indicate if the nurse may be an LPN or must be an RN. _____

   _____

4. List five places the graduate nurse may find specialized employment opportunities; indicate if the nurse employed in the setting will most often be an RN or LPN. _____ _____

   _____ _____

   _____

5. State the job-seeking skills the graduate will need to find employment. _____

6. Complete the following terms indicating methods for locating employment sites: The State _____ Service, N_____, B_____ B_____, and other sources, N_____ J_____, the I_____.

Part 4

Indicate if the following activities would be appropriate (A) or inappropriate (I).

1. _____ Planning to work a night shift, but keeping regular day hours on your off days to maintain a social life

2. _____ Taking a nap when you get a break during your night shift

3. _____ Bringing something interesting to do during your night shift to help you stay alert

4. _____ Keeping nursing records in different locations in the home so that all records will not be lost if a fire occurs in one room

5. _____ Placing a copy of professional documents in a file and keeping the originals in a safe deposit box

6. _____ Serving a period as a nurse intern to help the transition from student to practicing nurse

7. _____ Terminating all learning experiences with graduation from school; concentrating on practice

8. _____ Obtaining a permit to practice as a graduate nurse, if allowed in your state, before taking the nursing examination

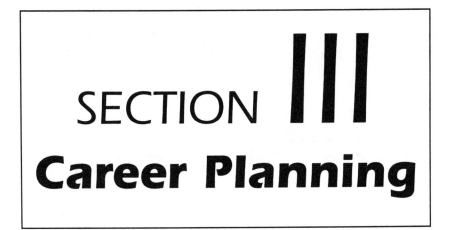

SECTION III
Career Planning

IDENTIFYING CAREER GOALS

With your choice to become an LPN/LVN you set goals to graduate from your nursing program and successfully complete the licensure exam. Determining the type of nursing career that is best for you is one of your most important goals. Career planning includes distinguishing between a job, which is a set of discrete tasks performed according to a job description for payment with emphasis on day to day employment, and a career, which is a pattern and sequence of positions which move you toward a career goal (Henderson and McGettigan, 1994).

Throughout your program you will have, or have had, experiences which will help you to determine career goals, the area of nursing in which you might like to work, and the contribution you want to make in health care delivery. As discussed in Chapter 99 of your text, the role of the LPN/LVN differs in each state and each facility. In addition, the settings in which the LPN might be employed vary from the traditional hospital position, to community positions such as the extended care facility, doctor's offices and clinics, and various other possibilities, including many specialty nursing positions.

In establishing career goals, the LPN student should explore the many roles they play in life and how their career will fit with these other roles. In addition, consider your personality, including your strengths, and your likes and dislikes. If you like a fast-paced environment with rapid patient turnover, you might prefer a same day procedure unit in a hospital or community to an extended care facility position. Consider if you enjoy working with children or adults, the elderly, or possibly terminally ill clients. These preferences will greatly influence your career choices. Once you determine the client population you wish to serve, you should consider your longterm goals. Would you like to work with a team of nurses, independently in home health, or as a clinic nurse with a physician? What are your financial needs? Does the position you want ultimately require additional education? Are you open for relocation? Ask yourself the question: Where would I like to be in 5 years? Then ask: What positions and activities will help me get there? Once you determine the position you will need to begin your career journey, seek available positions in that area.

FINDING AVAILABLE POSITIONS

Sources

Your text provides an excellent list of sources for locating employment sites. In addition to those listed, consider that professional organizations, state board of nursing, the schools of nursing, hospitals, and hospital association in your area or state may publish a newsletter or web page in which they post available positions for healthcare workers. Most important, remember the key concept mentioned in your text chapter that states that most positions are filled based on personal contacts. Your approach in seeking a nursing postion will be critical to your success in finding one.

Plan of Approach

Share your thoughts about, and your wants and desires for, a nursing position with your instructors and peers. In addition, ask questions as you rotate through various clinical experiences and facilities. Meet people and collect names of persons at various facilities. Networking is an important part of seeking employment and maintaining a nursing career. Networking begins before you enter your nursing program, continues through your program, and throughout your nursing career.

Remember to make your best first and subsequent impressions on your instructors, peers and professional contacts as you move through your nursing program. These will be persons you will contact for suggestions for employment sites, letters of reference, and opportunities to apply for positions. Establish a networking notebook. Enter the names and addresses, and phone numbers, professional cards if possible, of faculty, peers, and key persons at health care institutions you might wish to contact. Include e-mail addresses as well. Make an effort to contact persons in your notebook a least annually, even if just by sending a note related to your contact with them at their facility or in their class.

Ask faculty for permission to include them as possible references for employment positions and ask how they would wish to be contacted by persons seeking a reference for you. Your faculty are often well-connected to persons in the healthcare arena who would inform them of open positions and ask if faculty have suggestions for persons who would best fill these openings. Therefore a strong performance as a student nurse will result in a strong reference from faculty, facility nurses and administrators, and peers, to employers when you complete your program, as well as in the future.

In additional to personal contacts, systematically scan the journals, newspapers, bulletin boards, internet, and other sources posting nursing positions. Keeping abreast of available positions in nursing helps the student to refine career goals and focus job-seeking efforts upon graduation.

If relocation is an option, remember to explore opening in all areas of the country, and internationally, if interested. International and national journals, and the internet will be invaluable resources for broad job searches.

APPLICATION

The job application process provides the first official opportunity for you to present yourself as a potential employee. Again, first impressions are important, so from your initial phone call and letter of interest inquiring about position availability, through submission of your application and resume you want to create an impression of confidence, competence, and professionalism.

Letter of Interest

Your letter of interest and inquiry should be brief, clear, and specific to the position. The letter should include your full name and address above the date. You should address the letter to the individual specified in the advertisement or by your contact. If no specific person is indicated, and you are unable to determine the name of a specific nurse recruiter, address the letter to 'Dear Sir or Madam' or 'Dear personnel director.' Whenever possible, investigate to find the specific name of the person in charge of hiring nurses. A letter addressed to a specific person will give a more positive impression. Be careful to obtain correct spelling and current title.

The letter of interest should begin with a statement of interest in the position and should list the title of the position as advertised and the date and publication in which you found the advertisement. If you were informed of a possible position through a contact, state the individual's name and position and your understanding of the position opening as related to you by the individual.

In the next paragraph of the letter, you should briefly introduce yourself. You should present a summary of your qualifications for the position as compared to the employer's requirements as indicated in the advertisement. When possible, investigate the position requirements so you can use this information in your cover letter. As a student or recent graduate you should refer to any employment or educational experiences you have had that indicate your possession of skills related to the position. You might refer to your attached resume, or request an appointment to submit your application and to interview.

As stated previously, the letter of interest often presents a first impression of you to the potential employer. A powerful letter of interest presents a dynamic picture of the potential employee. A letter that is distinct catches the employer or personnel officer's attention which is important since there might be a large number of applicants. The way the letter is presented and organized, what it says and how the information is stated are all critical factors to the effectiveness of the letter.

Letterhead on your stationary or paper is impressive and can be prepared through most desk top publishing programs. You can include your address and phone numbers on the letterhead. Check with the library or computer department or media department if you don't have access to a computer, you may be able print your letterhead stationary in these locations, if you provide your own paper. Use a professional grade of paper and envelope.

The following are two sample advertisements for an LPN position, one in a hospital setting, and the other in a community setting. A sample letter of interest is presented for each advertisement.

Jillian L. Jacks
123 Jason Road
Albany, Georgia 32391

Home: (320) 555-4438
Voice mail: (321) 555-4428

April 30, 2001

Mrs. Ilinen Pauhl
Nurse Recruiter, Human Resources
ASAP Hospital
5454 Hospital Square
Denning, Delaware 23245

Dear Mrs. Pauhl:

The December edition of *PULSE* contained your advertisement for openings for LPNs in several areas in your institution. I am interested in a position in the Transitional Care Sub-Acute unit on the 7p to 7a shift. My qualifications are an excellent match for this position. I am enclosing a resumé for your consideration and would like to schedule a time to speak with you about the position.

I will graduate from the LPN program at Plum Technical Institute in May of this year. As a student I worked over 90 hours in a sub-acute unit with adult clients. Most of my time on this unit occurred during the evening and night shifts. Throughout my time in the sub-acute unit I performed multiple skills including urinary catheterization, diabetic testing and other skills which are listed on my resumé. In addition to my student experiences, I volunteered and served in several community campaigns in which I gave flu injections, performed blood pressure screening, and counseled clients on diet and exercise.

In addition to my nursing experience, I worked as a supervisor in a jewelry store for the two years prior to entering my nursing program, and over the past year while attending my nursing program. In this role I utilized skills in working as a team, providing information to consumers regarding the products we were selling, and in settling staff and customer disputes using tact and diplomacy. These people skills should be beneficial in the position you advertised particularly since your environment is one in which personal care is a priority.

I am dedicated to client care and excited about the prospect of assuming a position as an LPN in a caring environment. My resumé will provide additional information regarding my qualifications. I appreciate your consideration of my employment candidacy. Thank you for your consideration, and I look forward to meeting with you.

Sincerely,

Jillian Jacks

Enclosure

Medical Nursing: LPN

LPN positions for Med/Surg and Sub-Acute 7A-3P, includes weekend, days and evening shifts. PRN float for all shifts, Transitional Care Sub-Acute unit 7P-7A weekdays and weekends. Seeking experienced LPNs who would enjoy working in a mission driven environment where a committment to caring, personal care is a priority. Contact Human Resources Department, 812-555-1234, ASAP Hospital 5454 Hospital Square, Denning, Delaware.

(Upon calling human resources, you discovered that Mrs. Ilinen Pauhl is the nurse recruiter in the Human Resources department and will receive all applications for the LPN position)

Jillian L. Jacks
123 Jason Road
Albany, Georgia 32391

Home: (320) 555-4438
Voice mail: (321) 555-4428

October 31, 2001

Mrs. Debbie Broaden
Office Manager
Gastrointestinal Specialists, Inc.
5454 Hospital Square
Kenning, Florida 13245

Dear Mrs. Broaden:

I am interested in the LPN position you advertised in the November LPN Journal. As requested I am faxing my resumé which will reveal that my qualifications are a match for this position. I would also like to schedule a time to speak with you about the position.

I graduated from the LPN program at Plum Technical Institute in May of this year and have successfully obtained my licensure. As a student I worked over 90 hours in a clinic setting and also worked over 60 hours in a homeless clinic administering medications and assisting a nurse practitioner with physical exams. Throughout my time in both clinic settings I performed multiple skills including urinary catheterization, diabetic testing and other skills which are listed on my resumé. In addition to my student experiences, I volunteered and served in several community campaigns in which I gave flu injections, performed blood pressure screening, and counseled clients on diet and exercise.

In addition to my nursing experience, I worked in a jewelry store for the two years prior to entering my nursing program, and over the past year while attending my nursing program. In this role I utilized skills in working as a team, providing information to consumers regarding the products we were selling, and in settling staff and customer disputes using tact and diplomacy. These people skills should be beneficial in the position you advertised for your office.

I am dedicated to client care and excited about the prospect of assuming a position as an LPN in a caring environment. My resumé will provide additional information regarding my qualifications. I appreciate your consideration of my employment candidacy. Thank you for your consideration, and I look forward to meeting with you.

Sincerely,

Jillian Jacks

Enclosures

Nursing

LPN needed for a busy gastro practice with three doctors and a nurse practitioner. Clinical skills and good people skills required. Office experience desired. Good benefits. Fax resumé to 653-555-4938 or call Debbie at 653-555-3239. Salary negotiable with experience.

October 31, 2001

Mr. Donald Beard
Clinical Nurse Coordinator, Medical-Surgical Services
HIJ Hospital Systems
5454 Hospital Square
Kenning, Florida 13245

Dear Mr. Beard:

I will graduate from the LPN program at Plum Technical Institute in May of this year and anticipate successfully obtaining my license by July. I worked in your Medical unit during my clinical experiences as a student, and will complete a concentrated practicum in your unit this May. I enjoy working in your unit and am impressed by the quality of care provided to clients by you and your staff. I am interested in employment as an LPN at your hospital and particularly in your unit position. My experiences in your unit and throughout my program have helped me build skills that will help me to be a beneficial member of your staff.

As a student I worked over 100 hours in adult Medical-Surgical units. I also worked over 60 hours in a homeless clinic administering medications and assisting a nurse practitioner with physical assessments and procedures. In addition to my student clinical experiences, I volunteered and served in several community campaigns in which I gave flu injections, performed blood pressure screening, and counseled clients on diet and exercise.

In addition to my nursing experience, I worked in a jewelry store for the two years prior to entering my nursing program, and over the past year while attending my nursing program. In this role I utilized skills in working as a team, providing information to consumers regarding the products we were selling, and in settling staff and customer disputes using tact and diplomacy. These people skills would be beneficial as a member of the staff of your unit.

I am dedicated to client care and excited about the prospect of assuming a position as an LPN in a caring environment. My attached resumé will provide additional information regarding my qualifications. I will contact you on Monday, April 29th to schedule a time we might talk about staffing needs in your unit. If after reviewing my resumé you wish to contact me before Monday, please feel free to contact me at the above phone numbers. Thank you for your consideration of my employment candidacy, and I look forward to meeting with you.

Sincerely,

Jillian Jacks

Enclosures

APPLICATION (continued)

Many employers have a standard employment application. The length and content of the application may vary from facility to facility, but generally you must list your name, address, and phone number(s), educational background, work experience, and reasons for leaving past employment. In addition, some applications may request other information such as honors, awards, and your organizational affiliations, with emphases on offices held. Be truthful and thorough. Take great effort to supply accurate dates of graduation, degree names, dates of employment, and names of places employed, as well as names of your immediate supervisors. Answer all questions on the application, including placing the letters 'N/A' in spaces for questions that are not applicable to you or optional questions that you choose not to answer.

Keep a record of your activities, experiences, and honors with accurate dates and names. This record should start with high school and proceed through your time in your nursing program. Keep this notebook with you when you go to a facility to complete an application to assure accuracy of information. Update the notebook monthly as needed to promote the accuracy of the application and the resumé.

RESUMÉ

The resumé should be a succinct but thorough picture of your qualifications for an LPN position. You should develop a resumé that includes all of your experiences and activities, then adapt the resumé as needed for the position for which you are applying. The resumé should be two pages maximum, although one page is preferable. You may use a reverse chronological organization with the most recent experiences first, or group activities as full time, part time, and volunteer work, and formal or informal education. Use action verbs when describing your activities in your work, school, or organizational positions — "administered medications," "developed a plan for client assessment by nurse aides" The format and content of the resumé may vary but generally should include:

— Your full name, address with zip code, phone number(s) —indicate if home or office number, and fax or e-mail address if desired for communication.

— Professional goal or objective (optional) this brief statement should be tailored for the position and should indicate how well your professional goals match the mission or philosophy of the organization (the organizational goal and philosophy can be researched or may be stated in the advertisement).

— Education—formal, include the date of graduation or dates or attendance, the title of the degree or certification, and educational major/major classes attended if space is available. -Informal—As a student, workshops and classes/clinical experiences may fill this section.

— Work Experience—begin with experiences related to the job position, then experiences that are not directly related. Subdivide experiences by dates, listing fulltime first, then part time positions, then voluntary positions (important as a student). Emphasize duties in each position that resulted in development of skills needed to perform the desired job position.

— Skills—emphasize those skills you possess that would make you an asset as an employee, particularly those that make you unique or particularly well-qualified for the position.

— Licensure and Certifications—use full names of the license/certification and the organizations granting the license or certification, including abbreviations.

— Honors and awards—clearly identify the source of the award and reason for receiving award.

— Organizational memberships/offices held—include dates of membership and span of time office was held. If space allows, include any major accomplishment gained during your span in office or your membership activities.

— References list if space available or state "available upon request"

Include a variety of references from your educational, work, and volunteer experiences. Add a personal reference if desired. Choose an individual who can focus on your character and your organizational and people skills. Prescreen all references you wish to list. Ask the individual what type of reference they would provide if queried. Request permission to list the individual as a reference, and obtain the correct address and phone number by which the individual would like to be contacted.

The following is a sample of a resumé format followed by a sample resumé adapted for the position discussed with the letter of interest. Note that order of sections may vary and inclusion of an objective is optional.

<Name>
<Address> • *<City, State, Zip>* • *<Telephone>*

Objective

Use the "Section Heading" button to create additional sections in your resumé (Objective, Education, etc). Use the "Small Caps" and "Italics" buttons to add visual interest as shown below.

Experience

Title, Applicable Date(s)

ORGANIZATION NAME

RESPONSIBILITIES AND ACCOMPLISHMENTS.

Title, Applicable Date(s)

ORGANIZATION NAME

RESPONSIBILITIES AND ACCOMPLISHMENTS.

Education

INSTITUTION NAME

DEGREE, MAJOR AND YEAR

HONORS, RELATED ACTIVITIES, ACCOMPLISHMENTS.

INSTITUTION NAME

DEGREE, MAJOR AND YEAR

HONORS, RELATED ACTIVITIES, ACCOMPLISHMENTS.

Skills

• BULLETS MAY BE USED HERE TO CREATE AN ATTRACTIVE LIST OF SKILLS.

Advertisement—LPN needed for a busy gastro practice with three doctors and a nurse practitioner. Clinical skills and good people skills required. Office experience desired. Good benefits. Fax resumé to 653-555-4938 or call Debbie at 653-555-3239.

Jillian L. Jacks
123 JASON ROAD
ALBANY, GEORGIA 32391

HOME: (320) 555-4438
VOICE MAIL: (321) 555-4428

Objective

To work as an LPN in an ambulatory care setting as a member of a team of healthcare providers serving a population of clients undergoing diagnostic procedures for gastric conditions.

Employment

Nurse Tech   1998–1999
Marchal Hospital, Burbank, CA
Obtained vital signs, provided hygienic care, and performed bedside testing, such as glucose testing, on a group of 10 patients as a member of a nursing team.

Nursing Assistant   Present
St. Paul Homeless Clinic, Jelies, CA
Assisted Nurse practitioner with assessments and procedures such as pelvic examinations, wound dressing changes. Developed a teaching plan for teen clients on dressing changes.

EDUCATION

LPN Diploma   1999 (pending)
Plum Technical Institute,   Denene, CA
Major: Practical Nursing
Minor: Biology (15 extra hours taken)
Activities: Medical-Surgical Nursing—120 hours in adult care settings, administering medications, changing dressings, and performing diagnostic tests such as blood glucose and stool guaiac tests.

Diploma   1996
Bell High School,   Denene, CA
Major: General High school curriculum
Minor: Advanced biology and microbiology courses taken
Activities: Worked with school nurse in infirmary, assisted in cataloging supplies and with minor procedures such as bandaging wounds

SKILLS
- Client Assessment—vital signs
- Blood glucose monitoring
- Stool guaiac
- IV fluid monitoring
- Intake and output monitoring

REFERENCES: *upon request*

INTERVIEW

Great! you've been scheduled for an interview. Now, you must concentrate on presenting yourself as competent and confident, and focused. Your appearance should be professional. Dress appropriately. Clothing should be professional, comfortable and clean. The traditional black or blue suit is still a good choice; however, fashion in the business world has expanded to include suits or jacket sets with tasteful colors. Extremes should be avoided in clothing, jewelry perfume, and hair styles. Jewelry and make-up should reflect the image you expect to portray in your professional environment.

Be on time! It is better to be a few minutes early, since this allows you to compose yourself prior to the interview. Find the location of the interview in advance and allow for traffic delays or other problems that might delay you. If you are unavoidably delayed or must cancel your interview, *call as soon as possible and speak with the interviewer in person.* Ask to reschedule the interview as soon as possible.

Be prepared to respond to any questions honestly. Be aware, however, that employers have legal restrictions on the type of questions they are entitled to ask. Personal information such as whether or not you are married or have children should not be asked in the interview process. However, you may be asked if there is anything that may impact your ability to perform your duties or work the hours assigned to you. You may choose to volunteer information concerning your marital status or child care responsibilities and in some circumstances, it may be appropriate to do so. However, this is a decision each individual must make based on his or her circumstances. Remain calm and courteous. If you choose not to respond to a question, respectfully decline "I'd prefer not to answer that question, that is private information."

You might ask the purpose of the question and determine if there is other information you could supply that would satisfy the original purpose of the question.

Come prepared with questions of your own. For example, any questions about orientation, mentorship for each shift you will work, evaluation issues, salary issues, as well as continuing education requirements and opportunities could be addressed in this forum. If multiple positions are available in the setting, you should express a preference for the area you would like to work in and your willingness to accept alternate positions. Inquire about the time frame in which the decision for employment will be made.

Complete the interview by thanking your interviewer. Followup within a week with a thank you note: "I enjoyed my interview with you. I appreciate your considering me for a position at your facility and look forward to hearing from you." Use a card or write a note on nice personal stationary. Address your letter directly to the interviewer, and watch the spelling of the name and title of that individual.

PROFESSIONAL GROWTH AND CAREER ADVANCEMENT

Informal Education

Most institutions provide inservice education programs, or will finance your attendance of work-related conferences. Take advantage of special classes offered by your institution to keep personnel current with new techniques and procedures. Refresher courses may be offered by nursing schools or nursing organizations as well as other local organizations, such as the American Red Cross. Course length and content will vary, however, the purpose of such offerings is to update staff with information so that current technologies and advances are disseminated to nurses and other interested parties.

Formal Education

The opportunity to advance in nursing may include a decision to become a registered nurse through a diploma, associate degree or bachelor of science degree program.

Information on each type of program is readily available at libraries, nursing schools, and through nursing organizations.

PROFESSIONAL AFFILIATIONS

Your text discusses the benefits of belonging to professional organizations and lists many professional organizations available for the LPN/LVN. The following is a list of organizations and addresses:

Nursing Organizations

1. National Association for Practical Nurse Education and Service (NAPNES)
   254 West 31st Street, New York, NY 10001. NAPNES is the organization begun in 1941 to address issues relating to practical nurse education. Membership fees are paid annually and includes a subscription to the association's magazine, Journal of Practical Nursing.

2. National Federation of Licensed Practical Nurses (NFLPN) 214 S. Driver , P.O. Box 11038, Durham, NC 27703. NFLPN is the organization started in 1949 by licensed practical nurses and is the only organization composed entirely of licensed practical nurses and student practical nurses. Membership dues are paid once per year and includes a Subscription to their official magazine, The Journal of Nursing Care.

3. National League for Nursing, Inc. (NLN)—10 Columbus Circle, New York, NY 10019. NLN was established in 1952 by combining several organizations and committees. Members include individuals and agencies and there is a department for professional and practical nursing programs.

4. Your Alumni Association—Get involved with other graduates of your practical nursing program to stay connected with like-minded peers and to follow the progress of your nursing school. This also provides you with information on continuing education programs and other alumni activities.

Reference: Henderson, F. C. & McGettigan, B. O. (1994). *Managing Your Career in Nursing,* 2nd ed. New York: National League for Nursing Press. Pub. No. 14-2640.

Appendix

Below are the definitions of acronyms presented in this *Study Guide*. More may have been included here than in the textbook. Acronyms generally appear in the first chapter where they are introduced and sometimes are not repeated in any of the following chapters unless they are particularly relevant to the topics discussed in that chapter. For example, MI is introduced very early, as in the AIDS chapter. However, the acronym may be repeated in the chapter that actually describes the disorder (ie, MI is repeated in the cardiovascular chapter).

UNIT 1

Chapter 1

AIDS   acquired immunodeficiency syndrome
AJN   *American Journal of Nursing*
AMA   American Medical Association
ANA   American Nurses Association
HOSA   Health Occupations Students of America
ICN   International Council of Nurses
LPN   Licensed Practical Nurse
LVN   Licensed Vocational Nurse
NAPNES   National Association of Practical Nursing Education and Services
NCLEX   National Council Licensing Examination
NFLPN   National Federation of Licensed Practical Nurses
NLN   National League for Nursing
NSNA   National Student Nurses' Association
RN   Registered Nurse
VNS   Visiting Nurse Society
YMCA   Young Men's Christian Association
YWCA   Young Women's Christian Association

Chapter 2

AALPN   American Association of Licensed Practical Nurses
AD   associate degree
ANCC   American Nurses' Credentialing Center
CNA   Certified Nursing Assistant
e-mail   electronic mail
INC   International Nursing Center
NCLEX-PN   National Council Licensure Examination for Practical Nurses
NLN-CHAP   National League for Nursing—Community Health Accreditation Program
UAP   unlicensed assistive personnel

Chapter 3

CQI   continuous quality improvement
DRG   diagnosis-related group
ECF   extended care facility
HMO   health maintenance organization
HPRDA   Health Planning and Resources Development Act
ICF   intermediate care facility
IHS   Indian Health Services
JCAHO   Joint Commission on Accreditation of Healthcare Organizations
OSHA   Occupational Safety and Health Administration Act
PPO   preferred provider organization
RUG   resource utilization group
SSDI   Social Security Disability Insurance

Chapter 4

AHA   American Hospital Association
AMA   against medical advice, American Medical Association
CEU   continuing education unit
CNS   central nervous system
NAHC   National Association for Home Care
NCLEX-RN   National Council Licensing Examination for Registered Nurses
PSDA   Patient Self-Determination Act
UNOS   United Network of Organ Sharing

UNIT 2

Chapter 6

CHD   coronary heart disease
COPD   chronic obstructive pulmonary disease
HDL   high-density lipoprotein
HIV   human immunodeficiency virus
LDL   low-density lipoprotein
MI   myocardial infarction
MVA   motor vehicle accident
STD   sexually transmitted disease
WHO   World Health Organization

Chapter 7

ACS   American Cancer Society
ADAMHA   Alcohol, Drug Abuse, and Mental Health Administration
AHA   American Heart Association
ARC   American Red Cross
ATF   Alcohol, Tobacco and Firearms
BOH   Board of Health
CDC   Centers for Disease Control and Prevention
DOA   Department of Agriculture
DOH   Department of Health
EPA   Environmental Protection Agency
FDA   Food and Drug Administration
FQHC   Federally Qualified Healthcare
HRA   Health Resources Administration
HSA   Health Services Administration
MCHB   Maternal Child Health Bureau
MUA   medically underserved areas
NIH   National Institutes of Health
NIOSH   National Institute of Occupational Safety and Health
OMH   Office for Migrant Health
OTC   over-the-counter (drugs)
TTY   teletype
UN   United Nations
UNICEF   United National Children's Fund
USDHHS   US Department of Health and Human Services
USPHS   US Public Health Service
VNA   Visiting Nurse Association
WIC   Women, Infants, and Children (government program)

Chapter 8

LDS   Latter Day Saints, Church of Jesus Christ (Mormon)
RC   Roman Catholic

UNIT 3

Chapter 9

SO   significant other

UNIT 4

Chapter 15

DNA   deoxyribonucleic acid
H_2O   water
LLQ   left lower quadrant
LUQ   left upper quadrant
MASH   Mobile Army Surgical Hospital
μ   micron
RBC   red blood cell
RLQ   right lower quadrant
RUQ   right upper quadrant
WBC   white blood cell

Chapter 16

UV   ultraviolet (light, rays)

Chapter 17

ADH   antidiuretic hormone
ANP   atrial natriuretic peptide
ATP   adenosine triphosphate
CO_2   carbon dioxide
CSF   cerebrospinal fluid
ECF   extracellular fluid
HCl   hydrochloric acid
ICF   intracellular fluid
IVF   intravascular fluid
KCl   potassium chloride
mEq   milliequivalent
mL   milliliter
mL/d   milliliter per day
NaCl   sodium chloride salt
O_2   oxygen
pH   potential power of hydrogen ion

Chapter 18

ROM   range of motion

Chapter 19

ANS   autonomic nervous system
CNS   central nervous system
CSF   cerebrospinal fluid
EEG   electroencephalogram
kg   kilogram
PNS   peripheral nervous system

Chapter 20

ACTH   andrenocorticotropic hormone
ADH   antidiuretic hormone (vasopressin)
ANP   atrial natriuretic peptide
CRH   corticotropin-releasing hormone
FSH   follicle-stimulating hormone
HCG   human chorionic gonadotropin
ICSH   interstitial cell-stimulating hormone
GH   growth hormone
GRH, GHRH   growth-releasing hormone
GHIH   growth hormone-inhibiting hormone (somatostatin)
GNRH   gonadotropin-releasing hormone
LH   luteinizing hormone
MIH   melanocyte-inhibiting factor
MSH   melanocyte-stimulating hormone
PIH   prolactin-inhibiting hormone (dopamine)
PRH   prolactin-releasing hormone
PRL   prolactin, lactogenic hormone
PTH   parathormone/parathyroid hormone
TSH   thyroid-stimulating hormone
TRH   thyrotropin-releasing hormone
T_3   triiodothyronine
T_4   thyroxine

Chapter 22

AV   atrioventricular
BP   blood pressure
CO   cardiac output
HR   heart rate
LAD   left anterior descending artery
LCA   left coronary artery
LCX   left circumflex artery
LMCA   left main coronary artery
RAC   right coronary artery
SA   sinoatrial node
SV   stroke volume
SVR   systemic vascular resistance

Chapter 23

B cell   B lymphocyte
CO_2   carbon dioxide
Hgb, Hb   hemoglobin
Ig   immunoglobulin
O_2   oxygen
RBC   red blood cell
Rh   Rhesus, Rh factor, Rh negative or positive
T cell   T lymphocyte, T helper cells and other T cells
WBC   white blood cell

Chapter 24

Ab   antibody
Ig, IgG, IgM, IgA, IgE, IgD   immunoglobulin
TF   thymic factor
THF   thymic humoral factor

Chapter 25

CO   carbon monoxide
CO_2   carbon dioxide
ERV   expiratory reserve volume
H_2CO_3   carbonic acid
IRV   inspiratory reserve volume
O_2   oxygen
RV   residual volume
TLC   total lung capacity
TV   tidal volume
VC   vital capacity

Chapter 26

ATP   adenosine triphosphate
CHO   starch, carbohydrate
GI   gastrointestinal
HCl   hydrochloric acid

Chapter 27

ADH   antidiuretic hormone
ANP   atrial natriuretic peptide
BUN   blood urea nitrogen
cm   centimeter

Chapter 28

FSH   follicle-stimulating hormone
ICSH   interstitial cell-stimulating hormone

Chapter 29

ERT   estrogen replacement therapy
FSH   follicle-stimulating hormone
LH   luteinizing hormone

UNIT 5

Chapter 30

ADA   American Dietary Association
BMI   body mass index
C   kilocalorie
CHO   carbohydrate
DRI   dietary reference intake
EAR   estimated average requirement
ESADDI   estimated safe and adequate daily dietary intake
Fe   iron
GI   gastrointestinal
HDL   high-density lipoprotein
HFCS   high-fructose corn syrup
IF   intrinsic factor
Kcal   kilocalorie
LDL   low-density lipoprotein
NE   niacin equivalent
PCM   protein-calorie malnutrition
PKU   phenylketonuria
RDA   Recommended Dietary Allowance
RE   retinol equivalent
REE   resting energy expenditure
TE   tocopherol equivalent
UL   tolerable upper intake level
USDA   US Department of Agriculture

Chapter 32

FF   force fluid
G tube   gastrostomy tube
I & O   intake and output

IV   intravenous
J tube   jejunal tube
Na   sodium
Ng   nasogastric tube
NPO   nothing by mouth, nil peros
PEG   percutaneous endoscopic gastrostomy
STAT   immediately, at once
TPN   total parenteral nutrition

UNIT 6

Chapter 34

ADL   activities of daily living
CC   chief complaint

Chapter 35

EB   as evidenced by...
NANDA   North American Nursing Diagnosis Association
NCP   nursing care plan
POC   plan of care
PRN   as needed, pro re nata
R/T   related to...

Chapter 37

APIE   assessment, plan, intervention, evaluation
DAPE   data, assessment, plan, evaluation
DAR   data, action, response
CBE   charting by exception
MAR   medication administration record
MDS   minimum data set
MIS   Medical Information System
PIE   plan, intervention, evaluation
RAP   resident assessment protocol
RIE   recorded in error
SOAP   subjective, objective assessment, analysis, plan
SOAPIER   subjective, objective assessment, plan, intervention, evaluation, revision

Chapter 38

ASU ambulatory surgical unit
CCU coronary care unit
CDU chemical dependency unit
CSR central supply room
CSS central service supply
ECC emergency care center
ECF extended care facility
ECG electrocardiogram
ED Emergency department
EEG electroencephalogram
EMG electromyogram
ENT ear, nose, throat
ER emergency room
GI gastrointestinal
GU genitourinary
GYN gynecology
ICU intensive care unit
MRI magnetic resonance imaging
NEURO neurology
NICU newborn (neonatal) intensive care unit
OB obstetrics
OPD outpatient department
OPS outpatient surgery
OR operating room
ORTHO orthopedics
OT occupational therapy
PACU postanesthesia care unit
PEDS pediatrics
PICU pediatric intensive care unit
PSYCH psychiatry
PT physical therapy
REHAB rehabilitation
RT respiratory therapy
SCU special care unit
SDSU same-day surgery unit
SNF skilled nursing facility

Chapter 39

CPR cardiopulmonary resuscitation
DMAT disaster medical assistance team
MSDS Material Safety Data Sheet
OSHA Occupational Safety and Health Administration (Act)
RACE rescue, alert/alarm, confine, extinguish fire
START simple triage and rapid treatment (system)

Chapter 40

AIDS acquired immunodeficiency syndrome
ECHO enteric cytopathogenic human orphan (syndrome)

HIV human immunodeficiency virus
MRSA methicillin-resistant *Staphylococcus aureus*
TB tuberculosis
VRE vancomycin-resistant enterococci

Chapter 41

CDC Centers for Disease Control and Prevention
PPE personal protective equipment

Chapter 42

BBP blood-borne pathogens
CDC Centers for Disease Control and Prevention
HICPAC Hospital Infection Control Practices Advisory Committee
IV intravenous
TB tuberculosis

Chapter 43

ABCDE Airway and cervical spine, breathing, circulation and bleeding, disability, expose and examine
ACLS advanced cardiac life support
AED automated external defibrillator
AVPU alert, responds to verbals, responds to pain, unresponsive
BLS, BCLS basic (cardiac) life support
CNS central nervous system
CPR cardiopulmonary resuscitation
ED emergency department
EMS Emergency medical service
LOC level of consciousness
MAST military antishock trousers
MUA motor vehicle accident
PERRLA+C pupils equal, round, react to light, accommodation OK and coordinated
RICE rest, ice, compression, elevation
SIDS sudden infant death syndrome
SIRES stabilize, identify toxin, reverse effect, eliminate toxin, support
SUB Q subcutaneous (under the skin)

Chapter 46

Ap apical
A-R apical radial (pulse)
Ax axillary

BP   blood pressure
BPM   beats per minute
C   Celsius
DBP   diastolic blood pressure
F   Fahrenheit
HR   heart rate
I & O   intake and output
MAP   mean arterial pressure
PO   By mouth (per os)
R, PR   rectal, per rectum
SBP   systolic blood pressure
TPR   temperature, pulse, and respiration
VS   vital signs

Chapter 47

CO$_2$ carbon dioxide
CT   computed tomography
ECG   electrocardiogram
EEG   electroencephalogram
LOC   level of consciousness
LP   lumbar puncture
MRI   magnetic resonance imaging
O$_2$ oxygen
PET   positron emission tomography
PMI   point of maximum impulse

Chapter 48

AROM   actual range of motion
CPM   continuous passive motion
OOB   out of bed
PROM   passive range of motion
ROM   range of motion

Chapter 51

BM   bowel movement
I & O   intake and output
SP   suprapubic (catheter)
SSE   soap suds enema
TWE   tap water enema
UTI   urinary tract infection

Chapter 52

cc   cubic centimeter
C & S   culture and sensitivity

GI   gastrointestinal
I & O   intake and output
IV   intravenous
mL   milliliter
O & P   ova (eggs) and parasites
UA   urinalysis

Chapter 53

ACE   all cotton elastic
CMS   color, motion, sensitivity
TED   thromboembolytic disease (socks)

Chapter 55

AHCPR   Agency for Health Care Policy and Research
JCAHO   Joint Commission on Accreditation of Healthcare Organizations
PCA   patient-controlled analgesia
TENS   transcutaneous electrical nerve stimulation

Chapter 56

BP   blood pressure
CBC   complete blood count
ECG   electrocardiogram
I & O   intake and output
IV   intravenous
NPO   nothing by (per) mouth (os)
O$_2$ oxygen
OR   operating room
PACU   postanesthesia care unit
PAR   postanesthesia recovery (room)
RR   recovery room
TCDB   turn, cough, deep breathe
UA   urinalysis
VS   vital signs

Chapter 57

CSR   central supply room
CSS   central sterile supply
OR   operating room

Chapter 59

AD   advance directive
CPR   cardiopulmonary resuscitation
DNH   do not hospitalize
DNI   do not intubate
DNR   do not resuscitate
EEG   electroencephalogram
IV   intravenous
PSDA   Patient Self-Determination Act

Chapter 60

cc   cubic centimeter
G, g, gm   gram
gr   grain
gtt   drop
kg   kilogram
L   liter
mg   milligram
mL   milliliter
oz   ounce
%   percent
U   unit

Chapter 61

CNM   Certified Nurse Midwife
DDS   dentist (Doctor of Dental Surgery)
DO   Doctor of Osteopathy
DEA   Drug Enforcement Agency
DVM   Doctor of Veterinary Medicine
FDA   Food and Drug Administration
MD   Medical Doctor
NF   National Formulary
NIH   National Institutes of Health
NP   Nurse Practitioner
OTC   over-the-counter
PDR   *Physician's Desk Reference*
RPh   Registered Pharmacist
TO   telephone order
USD   United States Dispensary
USP   United States Pharmacopoeia
VO   verbal order
WWW   World Wide Web

Chapter 62

ACE   angiotensin-converting enzyme (inhibitors)
ANS   autonomic nervous system
ASA   aspirin (acetylsalicylic acid)

b.i.d.   twice a day
CA   cancer
C & S   culture and sensitivity
CNS   central nervous system
DM   dextromethorphan
GI   gastrointestinal
HCl   hydrochloric acid
HS   at bedtime (hour of sleep)
MOM   Milk of Magnesia
MS   morphine sulfate
NSAID   nonsteroidal anti-inflammatory drug
OTC   over-the-counter
PCN   penicillin
PPF   plasma protein fraction
PRN   as needed
PT   prothrombin time
PTT   partial thromboplastin time
QD   every day
q.i.d.   four times a day
SO$_4$ sulfate
SSKI   saturated solution of potassium iodide
t.i.d.   three times a day

Chapter 63

D$_5$W5%   dextrose in sterile water
D$_5$½NS5%   dextrose in half-normal saline (0.45% NS)
D$_5$NS5%   dextrose in normal saline (0.9% NS)
DRF   drip rate factor
GT   gastrostomy (tube)
gtt   drops
HS   at bedtime (hour of sleep)
ID   intradermal
IM   intramuscular
IV   intravenous
IVPB   intravenous piggyback
JT   jejunostomy tube
MAR   medication administration record
mg   milligram
mL   milliliter
NaCl   sodium chloride
NG   nasogastric
NS   normal saline (0.9% NaCl)
OD   right eye
OS   left eye
OU   both eyes
PICC   percutaneous intravenous central catheter
PO   by mouth (per os)
PRN   as needed
R, PR   rectum, by rectum
SL   sublingual
STAT   at once, immediately
subQ   subcutaneous
TD   transdermal
TPN   total parenteral nutrition
V   vagina

Chapter 64

BPM beats per minute
DES diethylstilbestrol
EDC estimated date of confinement
EDD estimated date of delivery
FAS fetal alcohol syndrome
FHT fetal heart tones
G, P gravida, para
HG hyperemesis gravidarum
OB obstetrics
RhoGAM anti-D gamma globulin
TPAL term, preterm, abortion, living

Chapter 65

AROM artificial rupture of membrane
BPM beats per minute
FHT fetal heart tones
RhoGAM anti-D gamma globulin
SROM spontaneous rupture of membranes
SVE sterile vaginal examination

Chapter 66

G6PD glucose-6-phosphate dehydrogenase
PKU phenylketonuria
SIDS sudden infant death syndrome

Chapter 67

Ab abortion
AFP α-fetoprotein
CD cesarean deliver, chemical dependency
CPD cephalopelvic disproportion
CVS chorionic villus sample
D & C dilation and curettage
FBP fetal biophysical profile
FHT fetal heart tones
GDM gestational diabetes mellitus
HELLP hemolysis, elevated liver enzymes, low platelet count
Hg mercury
HG hyperemesis gravidarum
IV intravenous
LOP left occiput posterior
LS lecithin/sphingomyelin (ratio)
MgSO$_4$ magnesium sulfate
MSAFP maternal serum α-fetoprotein

NPO nothing by mouth
NST nonstress test
OCT oxytocin challenge test
OP occiput posterior
PIH pregnancy-induced hypertension
PROM premature rupture of membranes
PUBS percutaneous umbilical blood sample
RhoGAM anti-D gamma globulin
ROP right occiput posterior
STD sexually transmitted disease
SVE sterile vaginal examination
US ultrasound

Chapter 68

AGA appropriate for gestational age
AIDS acquired immunodeficiency syndrome
CMV cytomegalovirus
DS Down syndrome
EF erythroblastosis fetalis
FAS fetal alcohol syndrome
H$_2$O water
HIV human immunodeficiency virus
HSV herpes simplex virus
LBW low birth weight
LGA large for gestational age
NEC necrotizing enterocolitis
NICU newborn intensive care unit
PO$_2$ pressure of oxygen
PKU phenylketonuria
PT preterm
RDS respiratory distress syndrome
SGA small for gestational age
SIDS sudden infant death syndrome
VLBW very low birth weight

Chapter 69

AIDS acquired immunodeficiency syndrome
CMV cytomegalovirus
FTA-ABS fluorescent treponemal antibody absorption (test)
HIV human immunodeficiency virus
HPV human papillomavirus
HSV herpes simplex virus
IUD intrauterine device
IVF in vitro fertilization
PID pelvic inflammatory disease
Pap Papanicolaou (test)
RPR rapid plasma reagin (test)
STD sexually transmitted disease
VDRL Venereal Disease Research Laboratory

Chapter 70

DTP diphtheria, tetanus, pertussis
I & O intake and output
IV intravenous
LP lumbar puncture
MMR measles, mumps, rubella
NPO nothing by mouth
OFC occipital-frontal circumference
PICC percutaneous intravenous central catheter
TPN total parenteral nutrition
URI upper respiratory infection

Chapter 71

ALL acute lymphocytic (lymphoid) leukemia
AML acute myelogenous leukemia
ASO antistreptolysin O (titer)
AV atrioventricular (defect, shunt)
BRAT banana, rice cereal, applesauce, toast (diet)
CF cystic fibrosis
CNS central nervous system
CPR cardiopulmonary resuscitation
CPT chest physiotherapy
CT computed tomography
DH diaphragmatic hernia
DTP diphtheria, tetanus, pertussis
ECG electrocardiogram
ED emergency department
EEG electroencephalogram
ESR erythrocyte sedimentation rate
FTT failure to thrive
GI gastrointestinal
HUS hemolytic uremic syndrome
I & O intake and output
ITP idiopathic thrombocytopenic purpura
IV intravenous
LOC level of consciousness
LTB laryngotracheobronchitis
MMR measles, mumps, rubella
MRI magnetic resonance imaging
MTX methotrexate
NPO nothing by mouth
O & P ova (eggs) and parasites
OFC occipital-frontal circumference
ORS oral rehydration solution
PDA patent ductus arteriosus
PE polyethylene (tubes)
PKU phenylketonuria
PET positron emission tomography
PIA prolonged infantile apnea
RBC red blood count, red blood cell
RSV respiratory syncytial virus
SIDS sudden infant death syndrome
SGA small for gestational age
T & A tonsillectomy and adenoidectomy
TPN total parenteral nutrition

URI upper respiratory infection
WBC white blood count, white blood cell

Chapter 72

AN anorexia nervosa
CUC chronic ulcerative colitis
IBD inflammatory bowel disease
IDDM insulin-dependent diabetes mellitus
JRA juvenile rheumatoid arthritis
NSAID nonsteroidal anti-inflammatory drug
REM rapid eye movement (sleep)
RP retinitis pigmentosa
STD sexually transmitted disease

Chapter 73

ADDH attention deficit disorder with hyperactivity
ADHD attention deficit-hyperactivity disorder
ADL activities of daily living
AFP α-fetoprotein
AIDS acquired immunodeficiency syndrome
ALT alanine aminotransferase
AST aspartate aminotransferase
CNS central nervous system
COA children of alcoholics
CP cerebral palsy
CPK creatine phosphokinase
EEG electroencephalogram
FAS fetal alcohol syndrome
FTT failure to thrive
HIV human immunodeficiency virus
II intellectual impairment
IQ intelligence quotient
MBD minimal brain dysfunction
MD muscular dystrophy
SLD specific (special) learning disability

Chapter 74

AgNO₃ silver nitrate
CEA cultured epithelial autografts
DTIC dimethyltriazenoimidazole carboxamine (dacarbazine)
mm Hg millimeters of mercury
mL/kg milliliters per kilogram (of body weight)
I & O intake and output
IV intravenous
NPO nothing by mouth
PRN as needed
ROM range of motion

SPF   sun protective factor
TBSA   total body surface area
TPN   total parenteral nutrition
UV   ultraviolet (light, rays)

Chapter 75

C   chloride
Ca   calcium
CNS   central nervous system
CO$_2$ carbon dioxide (plasma CO$_2$ = carbonic acid)
ECF   extracellular fluid
GI   gastrointestinal
ICF   intracellular fluid
I & O   intake and output
IV   intravenous
K   potassium
mEq/L   milliequivalents per liter
Mg   magnesium
mg/dL   milligrams per deciliter
Na   sodium
P   phosphorous
pH   hydrogen ion concentration
PO$_4$ phosphate

Chapter 76

AEA   above elbow amputation
AKA   above knee amputation
AS   ankylosing spondylitis
BEA   below elbow amputation
BKA   below knee amputation
CK   creatine kinase
CMS   color (circulation), motion (movement), sensitivity (sensation)
CPM   continuous passive motion
DJD   degenerative joint disease
DVT   deep vein thrombosis
EF   external fixation
EMG   electromyogram
ESR   erythrocyte sedimentation rate
IVD   intervertebral disk disease
LD   lumbar decompression
NASAID   nonsteroidal anti-inflammatory drug
ORIF   open reduction, internal fixation
PCA   patient-controlled analgesia
RA   rheumatoid arthritis
RF   rheumatoid factor
ROM   range of motion
SLE   systemic lupus erythematosus
TENS   transcutaneous (transdermal) electrical nerve stimulation
THA   total hip arthroplasty (replacement)
TLSO   thoracic-lumbar-sacral orthosis (brace)
TMJ   temporomandibular joint (disorder)

Chapter 77

ADL   activities of daily living
ALS   amyotrophic lateral sclerosis (Lou Gehrig's disease)
ATM   acute transverse myelitis
CHT   closed head trauma
CNS   central nervous system
CSF   cerebrospinal fluid
CT   computed tomography
EEG   electroencephalogram
HD   Huntington's disease
HZ   herpes zoster
ICP   intracranial pressure
IICP   increasing (increased) intracranial pressure
LOC   level of consciousness
LP   lumbar puncture (spinal tap)
MAO   monoamine oxidase
MG   myasthenia gravis
MRI   magnetic resonance imaging
MS   multiple sclerosis
PD   Parkinson's disease
PET   positron emission tomography
SE   status epilepticus
TPN   total parenteral nutrition

Chapter 78

ACE   angiotensin-converting enzyme
ACTH   adrenocorticotropic hormone
ADA   American Diabetes Association
ADH   antidiuretic hormone (vasopressin)
BIDS   bedtime insulin and daytime sulfonylurea (regimen)
BR   buffered regular (insulin)
FPG   fasting plasma glucose
FSH   follicle-stimulating hormone
GDM   gestational diabetes mellitus
GH   growth hormone
GSH   glycosylated hemoglobin
GTT   glucose tolerance test
IDDM   insulin-dependent diabetes mellitus
IFG   impaired fasting glucose
IGT   impaired glucose tolerance
I & O   intake and output
LH   luteinizing hormone
NHS   nonketotic hyperosmolar state
NIDDM   non–insulin-dependent diabetes mellitus
OGTT   oral glucose tolerance test
PTH   parathormone
RAIU   radioactive iodine uptake (test)
SIADH   syndrome of inappropriate antidiuretic hormone
SMBG   self-monitoring of blood glucose
STH   somatotropic hormone
TFT   thyroid function test
TSH   thyroid-stimulating hormone
VMA   vanillylmandelic acid

Chapter 79

EEG   electroencephalogram
ENG   electronystagmogram
ERG   electroretinogram
IOL   intraocular lens implant
MRI   magnetic resonance imaging
OD   Doctor of Optometry, oculus dexter (right eye)
OS   oculus sinister (left eye)
OU   both eyes
OSHA   Occupational Safety and Health Administration (Act)
RGP   rigid gas-permeable (contact lenses)

Chapter 80

AICD   automatic implantable cardioverter-defibrillator
AST   aspartate aminotransferase
BP   blood pressure
CAD   coronary artery disease
CC   cardiac catheterization
CCU   coronary care unit
CHF   congestive heart failure
CICU   coronary intensive care unit
CPK   creatine phosphokinase
CPM   continuous passive motion
CPR   cardiopulmonary resuscitation
CVA   cerebrovascular accident (stroke)
DVT   deep vein thrombosis
ECG   electrocardiogram
EPS   electrophysiology study
HTN   hypertension
ICD   implantable cardioverter-defibrillator
I & O   intake and output
LDH   lactic dehydrogenase
MI   myocardial infarction (heart attack)
NS   nuclear scan
PE   pulmonary embolism
PROM   passive range of motion
PT   prothrombin time
PTCA   percutaneous coronary angioplasty
PTT   partial thromboplastin time
t-PA   tissue plasminogen activator
TPN   total parenteral nutrition
VV   varicose veins

Chapter 81

ABO   A, B, O blood types
ALL   acute lymphoblastic leukemia
AML   acute myelogenous leukemia
APTT   activated partial thromboplastin time
BMT   bone marrow transplant

CBC   complete blood count
CLL   chronic lymphocytic leukemia
CML   chronic myelogenous leukemia
DIC   disseminated intravascular coagulation
diff   differential (blood cell count)
ESR   erythrocyte sedimentation rate
FFP   fresh frozen plasma
HCT   hematocrit
HD   Hodgkin's disease
Hgb   hemoglobin
IG   immunoglobulins
ITP   idiopathic thrombocytopenic purpura
IV   intravenous
IVIG   intravenous immune globulin
NHL   non-Hodgkin's lymphoma
PBSC   peripheral blood stem cell
PPF   plasma protein fraction
PT   prothrombin time
PTT   partial thromboplastin time
RBC   red blood cell (erythrocyte)
T & C   type and crossmatch
WBC   white blood cell

Chapter 82

ACS   American Cancer Society
AFP   α-fetoprotein
BCNU   bischloroethylnitrosourea
BMT   bone marrow transplant
BRM   biologic response modifier
BSE   breast self-examination
CA   cancer, carcinoma
CAF   Cytoxan, Adriamycin, fluorouracil
CCNU   lomustine
CEA   carcinoembryonic antigen
CHOP   cyclophosphamide, doxorubicin, vincristine, prednisone
CMF   Cytoxan, methotrexate, fluorouracil
EBRT   external beam radiation therapy
DTIC   dimethyltriazenoimidazole carboxamide (dacarbazine)
5-FU   5-fluorouracil
HGF   hematopoietic growth factor
HCG   human chorionic gonadotropin
Ifex   ifosfamide
IFN   interferon
ILS   interleukins
NCI   National Cancer Institute
ONS   Oncology Nursing Society
Pap test   Papanicolaou's test
PIC   peripheral indwelling catheter
PICC   peripherally inserted central catheter
PSA   prostate-specific antigen
TSE   testicular self-examination
TSPA, TESPA   thiotepa
USDHHS   US Department of Health and Human Services

Chapter 84

AIDS acquired immunodeficiency syndrome
ARD AIDS-related dementia
B cells B lymphocytes (bone marrow)
CDC Centers for Disease Control and Prevention
DDC dideoxycytidine
DDI didanosine (Videx)
ELISA enzyme-linked immunosorbent assay
HIV human immunodeficiency virus
INH isoniazid
IV intravenous
KS Kaposi's sarcoma
PCP *Pneumocystis carinii* pneumonia
PCR polymerase chain reaction
T cells T lymphocytes (thymus T-helper cells)
ZDU zidovudine (formerly AZT)

Chapter 85

ABG arterial blood gas
ARDS adult respiratory distress syndrome
BCG bacille Calmette-Guérin
COLD chronic obstructive lung disease
COPD chronic obstructive pulmonary disease
CPAP continuous positive airway pressure
CPT chest physiotherapy
C & S culture and sensitivity
CT computed tomography, chest tube
CWSD closed water-seal drainage
DNS deviated nasal septum
flu influenza
INH isoniazid
IPPB intermittent positive pressure breathing
IS incentive spirometer
LS lung scan (scintiscan)
mm Hg millimeters of mercury
MRI magnetic resonance imaging
PaCO$_2$ partial pressure of carbon dioxide
PaO$_2$ partial pressure of oxygen
PCP *Pneumocystis carinii* pneumonia
PD postural drainage
PFT pulmonary function test
pH hydrogen ion concentration
PZA pyrazinamide
RBC red blood cell
ROM range of motion
RT respiratory therapy
SA sleep apnea
SOB shortness of breath
TB tuberculosis
TCDB turn, cough, deep breathe
URI upper respiratory infection

Chapter 86

ABG arterial blood gas
ARDS adult respiratory distress syndrome
CO$_2$ carbon dioxide
COLD chronic obstructive lung disease
COPD chronic obstructive pulmonary disease
CPAP continuous positive airway pressure, hyperbolic oxygenation
HBO hyperbaric oxygen
IPPB intermittent positive pressure breathing
LPM liters per minute
NC nasal cannula
NRM non-rebreathing mask
O$_2$ oxygen
O$_2$ sat. oxygen saturation (%)
PPV positive pressure ventilator
PRM partial rebreathing mask
PSV pressure support ventilation
SIMV synchronized intermittent mandatory ventilation
SOB shortness of breath

Chapter 87

ALT alanine aminotransferase (serum)
AN anorexia nervosa
AP abdominal paracentesis
AST aspartate aminotransferase (serum)
BAS barium swallow
BE barium enema
BRM biologic response modifiers
CA 19-9 carbohydrate antigen 19-9
CDC Centers for Disease Control and Prevention
CEA carcinoembryonic antigen (assay)
CT computed tomography
CUC chronic ulcerative colitis
DTAD drain tube attachment device
EGD esophagogastroduodenoscopy
ERCP endoscopic retrograde cholangiopancreatic assay
ET Enterostomal Therapist
5-FU 5-fluorouracil
GA gastric analysis
GGT γ-glutamyl transpeptidase
GI gastrointestinal
H$_2$ histamine
HAV hepatitis A virus (infectious hepatitis)
HBV hepatitis B virus (serum hepatitis)
HCV hepatitis C virus (non-A, non-B hepatitis)
HDV hepatitis D virus
HEV hepatitis E virus
HSV herpes simplex virus
IL-2 interleukin-2
IV intravenous
I & O intake and output
IBD inflammatory bowel disease

LES lower esophageal sphincter
LFT liver function test
LGI lower GI (x-rays)
NPO nothing by (per) mouth (os)
NSAID nonsteroidal anti-inflammatory drug
O & P ova and parasites
RBC red blood cell
TAC time, amount, character
TMJ temporomandibular joint
TNM tumor size, (lymph) node involvement, metastasis
TPN total parenteral nutrition
UGI upper GI (x-rays)
US ultrasound

Chapter 88

AIDS acquired immunodeficiency syndrome
ARF acute renal failure
BPH benign prostatic hyperplasia (hypertrophy)
BUN blood urea nitrogen
CAPD continuous ambulatory peritoneal dialysis
C & S culture and sensitivity
CGN chronic glomerulonephritis
CMG cystometrogram
CRF chronic renal failure
ECHD extracorporeal hemodialysis
EMG electromyogram
ESRD end-stage renal failure
ESWL extracorporeal shock wave lithotripsy
HIV human immunodeficiency virus
IPV intravenous pyelogram
KUB kidney-ureter-bladder (x-ray)
PEMG perineal electromyogram
RAG right arm gortex
RBC red blood cell
RP retrograde pyelogram
SPC (SPUC) suprapubic (urethral) catheter
TURBT transurethral resection of a bladder tumor
UA urinalysis
UC urine culture
UPP urethral pressure profile
UTI urinary tract infection
WBC white blood cell

Chapter 89

ABP acute bacterial prostatitis
ARRP anatomic radical retropubic prostatectomy
BPH benign prostatic hyperplasia
CBP chronic bacterial prostatitis
NBP nonbacterial prostatitis
PSA prostate-specific antigen
TSE testicular self-examination
TURP transurethral resection of the prostate
UA/UC urinalysis/urine culture

Chapter 90

AC anteroposterior (repair)
ACS
AP
BSE breast self-examination
CA cancer
CMF Cytoxan, methotrexate, 5-fluorouracil (5-FU)
D & C dilation and curettage
DES diethylstilbestrol
DVT deep vein thrombosis
GYN gynecology
HPV human papillomavirus
HRT hormone replacement therapy
in situ in place
IUD intrauterine device
Pap Papanicolaou's test
PID pelvic inflammatory disease
PMS premenstrual syndrome
STD sexually transmitted disease
TSS toxic shock syndrome
US ultrasound

Chapter 91

ALF assisted living facility
LTC long-term care
TPN total parenteral nutrition
VA vulnerable adult

Chapter 92

AD Alzheimer's disease
ADL activities of daily living
ADRDA Alzheimer's Disease and Related Disorders Association
AIDS acquired immunodeficiency syndrome
ALT alanine aminotransferase
BPRS Brief Psychiatric Rating Scale
CT computed tomography
EEG electroencephalogram
FADL functional activities of daily living
HD Huntington's disease
IADL instrumental activities of daily living
ID identification
MID multi-infarct dementia
MRI magnetic resonance imaging
PET positron emission tomography
RPR rapid plasma reagin (test)
SDAT senile dementia of the Alzheimer's type
SPECT single photon emission computed tomography
VDRL Venereal Disease Research Laboratory

Chapter 93

ADL   activities of daily living
AH   auditory hallucinations
AIDS   acquired immunodeficiency syndrome
AP   assault precautions
APA   American Psychiatric Association
BPD   bipolar disorder
BPRS   Brief Psychiatric Rating Scale
CIC   Crisis Intervention Center
CNS   central nervous system
CT   computed tomography
DCH   District Court Hold
DISCUS   Dyskinesia Identification System Condensed User Scale
DSM-IV   *Diagnostic and Statistical Manual of Mental Disorders*, 4th edition
ECG   electrocardiogram
ECT   electroconvulsive therapy
EEG   electroencephalogram
EP   escape (elopement) precaution
EPSE   extrapyramidal side effects
ETOH   alcohol (ethanol)
GP/SP   general precautions/suicide precaution
HHA   Home Health Aide
HI   homicidal ideation
KELS   Kohlman Evaluation of Living Skills
LOC   level of consciousness
MAO   monoamine oxidase
MAOI   monoamine oxidase inhibitor
MI/CD   mentally ill/chemically dependent
MI & D   mentally ill and dangerous
MMPI   Minnesota Multiphasic Personality Inventory
MMSE   Mini Mental Status Examination
MRI   magnetic resonance imaging
NMSN   neuroleptic malignant syndrome
NSAID   nonsteroidal anti-inflammatory drug
OCD   obsessive-compulsive disorder
OT   occupational therapy
PADS   personal aggression (assault) device system
PCA   personal care attendant
PET   positron emission tomography
PD   provisional discharge
PTSD   post-traumatic stress disorder
REBT   Rational Emotive Behavior Therapy (RBT)
REM   rapid eye movement
SA   suicide attempt
SI   suicidal ideation
SIB   self-injurious behavior
SPECT   single photon emission computed tomography
SSDI   Social Security Disability Insurance
SSRI   selective serotonin reuptake inhibitor
SX   sexual (precautions)
SZ   seizure (precautions)
TAT   Thematic Apperception Test
TCD   transcranial Doppler
TD   tardive dyskinesia
T-hold   transportation hold

TR   therapeutic recreation
WBC   white blood cell
W/D   withdrawal
WHO   World Health Organization
VH   visual hallucinations

Chapter 94

AA   Alcoholics Anonymous
ACOA   Adult Children of Alcoholics (association)
APA   American Psychiatric Association
CD   chemical dependency
CNS   central nervous system
COA   children of alcoholics
$D_5\frac{1}{2}NS$ half-normal saline with 5% dextrose
DTs   delirium tremens
EEG   electroencephalogram
ETOH   alcohol (ethanol)
FAS   fetal alcohol syndrome
LSD   lysergic acid diethylamide
$MgSO_4$ magnesium sulfate
MI/CD   mentally ill/chemically dependent
MJ   marijuana ("weed")
NA   Narcotics Anonymous
NSAID   nonsteroidal anti-inflammatory drug
OTC   over-the-counter (drug)
PCP   phencyclidine hydrochloride ("angel dust")
RET   Rational Emotive Therapy
THC   tetrahydrocannabinol (cannabis)
W/D   withdrawal

Chapter 95

ADL   activities of daily living
ALS   amyotrophic lateral sclerosis
B & C   board and care
CF   cystic fibrosis
CHT   closed head trauma
CPM   continuous passive motion
CVA   cerebrovascular accident
ECF   extended care facility
FADL   functional activities of daily living
FES   functional electrical stimulation
HD   Huntington's disease
IADL   instrumental activities of daily living
ICF   intermediate care facility
ICU   intensive care unit
MI   myocardial infarction
MVA   motor vehicle accident
PM & R   physical medicine and rehabilitation
PROM   passive range of motion
ROM   range of motion
SNF   skilled nursing facility
TBI   traumatic brain injury

TENS   transcutaneous electrical nerve stimulation
UAP   unlicensed assistive personnel

PCA   patient-controlled analgesia
TENS   transcutaneous electrical nerve stimulation
WHO   World Health Organization

Chapter 96

ACS   ambulatory care sensitive
CHC   community health center
CHHA   Certified Home Health Aide
ECG   electrocardiogram
EHS   Employee Health Service
EMT   Emergency Medical Technician
FHC   Family Health Center
HCA   Health Care Assistant
HHA   Home Health Aide
HMO   health maintenance organization
IV   intravenous
NAHC   National Association for Home Care
NPO   nothing by mouth
PCA   personal care attendant
PCP   primary care provider
PHN   Public Health Nurse

Chapter 98

CLTC   certified in long-term care
D/C   discontinued/discharged
ECF   extended care facility
MAR   medication administration record
NFLPN   National Federation of Licensed Practical Nurses
NLN   National League for Nursing
SNF   skilled nursing facility
TO   telephone order
UAP   unlicensed assistive personnel
VO   verbal order
WWW   World Wide Web

Chapter 97

ABHR   Ativan, Benadryl, Haldal, Reglan
AIDS   acquired immunodeficiency syndrome
DNH   do not hospitalize
DNI   do not intubate
DNR   do not resuscitate
IV   intravenous
MOM   Milk of Magnesia
NHO   National Hospice Organization

Chapter 99

CAT   computer adaptive test
CEU   continuing education unit
ECF   extended care facility
NAPNES   National Association for Practical Nursing Education and Service
NCLEX   National Council Licensing Examination
NFLPN   National Federation of Licensed Practical Nurses
OSHA   Occupational Safety and Health Administration (Act)

Answer Key

CHAPTER 1

Part 1

1. C
2. A
3. A
4. B
5. A

Part 2

1. F New York
2. F Nursing history
3. T
4. F 19th century
5. T

Part 3

1. G
2. I
3. K
4. H
5. L
6. B
7. J
8. D
9. C
10. A
11. F
12. E

Part 4

2—1979	7—1909
5—1938	4—1955
8—1900	9—1893
12—1844	6—1914
1—1994	3—1966
10—1881	11—1873

CHAPTER 2

Part 1

1. Registered, licensed practical/vocational
2. Approved, accredited

3. Any two of the following: National organizations: National Association for Practical Nurse Education and Service (NAPNES), National Federation of Licensed Practical Nurses (NFLPN), American Association of Licensed Practical Nurses (AALPN), National League for Nursing-Community Health Accreditation Program (NLN-CHAP), Health Occupations Students of America (HOSA), and American Nurses Association (ANA); or state affiliates of national organizations; or international nursing organizations

Part 2

1. T
2. T
3. F

Part 3

Terms and definitions will vary based on student.

Part 4

1. Permissive licensure
2. Advanced practice
3. Theoretical framework

Part 5

1. Difficult, change
2. Illness
3. Approved, accredited
4. Teacher, leader, team member

Part 6

1. LPN/LVN
2. RN
3. LPN/LVN

Part 7

1. C
2. D
3. A

CHAPTER 3

Part 1

1. *Reform*
2. *Holistic*
3. *Quality Assurance*
4. *Financing*
5. *Complementary*

Part 2

1. Any two of the following: hospitals–acute care facilities, extended care facilities, community health services
2. Whole

Part 3

Response will vary with student, definitions in text.

Part 4

1. Advocacy
2. Medicaid
3. Consumer fraud
4. Capitation fee
5. JCAHO

Part 5

1. F
2. F
3. T
4. F

5. F
6. T
7. F
8. T
9. F
10. T

Part 6

1. D
2. H
3. G
4. F
5. A
6. I
7. B
8. J
9. E
10. C

Part 7

1. Both terms are used for prospective payment based on categories, DRGs are used in hospital or home care, RUG is used in nursing homes and ECFs.
2. Both federal programs, Medicaid states can individually regulate, whereas Medicare is federally managed (see pages 31–32 for more information).
3. In SNF 24-hour nursing care is provided under supervision of RN; in ICF 24-hour services are provided under the supervision of an LPN with RN as a consultant (see page 28).

CHAPTER 4

Part 1

1. 2
2. 3
3. 1
4. 4

Part 2

1. Legally, ethically
2. Ethical Standards of Healthcare

Part 3

Response will vary with student, definitions in text.

Part 4

1. Living will
2. Euthanasia
3. Liability
4. Assault
5. Informed consent

Part 5

1. T
2. F
3. T
4. F
5. F

Part 6

1. E
2. I
3. F
4. B
5. J
6. H
7. D
8. A
9. G
10. C

Part 7

1. Power versus vulnerability, boundary crossing, boundary violations or professional sexual misconduct
2. Any two of the following: directive to physicians, durable power of attorney for healthcare, or mental health advance declaration
3. Any two of the following: the hospitalized individual, mentally ill, mentally retarded, confused person, or older person

CHAPTER 5

Part 1

1. Hierarchy
2. Relationship, needs
3. Family, community

Part 2

1. Any three of the following: oxygen, water and fluids, food and nutrients, elimination of waste products, sleep and rest, activity and exercise, or sexual gratification
2. Security, safety

Part 3

1. C
2. E
3. D
4. B
5. A

Part 4

1. Hierarchy
2. Sexual gratification
3. Primary needs
4. Social needs

Part 5

1. C
2. B
3. C
4. A
5. B

CHAPTER 6

Part 1

1. B
2. D
3. A
4. B
5. C
6. B

Part 2

1. Metastasis
2. Osteoporosis
3. Stress
4. Antioxidants
5. Lifestyle factors

Part 3

1. D
2. A
3. B
4. B
5. C

Part 4

1. Any four of the following (see text for more details).
   Physical activity: participation enhances energy, reduces stress, and provides relaxation.
   Nutrition: proper nutrition reduces problems resulting from poor nutrition such as heart failure.
   Tobacco: smoking cessation has an immediate effect on the improvement of health.
   Alcohol and drugs: decreasing alcohol and drug abuse will decrease the accidents and homicides related to this abuse.
   Family planning and sexuality: appropriate measures can reduce infant mortality, pediatric problems, STDs, unwanted pregnancies, and pregnancy in teens and substance-abusing women.

Stress: stress management techniques can assist people to manage harmful stress.
Violence and abuse: conflict resolution and anger management programs may help reduce violence.

2. Teach pregnant women about and encourage: early prenatal care, avoidance of tobacco and alcohol, and dietary supplements of folic acid, avoidance of chickenpox and STDs, and using caution with household chemicals and cat litter.
   Instruct clients to follow a low-fat diet, adhere to screening recommendations for specific cancers, avoid overexposure to the sun, and refrain from smoking.

Part 5

1. B
2. A
3. B
4. D
5. D

CHAPTER 7

Part 1

1. 5
2. 3
3. 4
4. 1
5. 2

Part 2

1. Advocate, educator
2. Healthcare worldwide

Part 3

Responses will vary with student, definitions in text.

Part 4

1. Biohazardous
2. Ecology
3. Plumbism
4. Consortium
5. Primary healthcare

Part 5

1. F
2. T
3. F
4. F
5. T

Part 6

1. B
2. A
3. E
4. C
5. D

Part 7

1. C
2. B
3. B

CHAPTER 8

Part 1

1. Y
2. Y
3. N
4. Y
5. Y

Part 2

1. Not always
2. Culturally influenced components

Part 3

1. F
2. F
3. T
4. F
5. T

Part 4

1. Rituals
2. Beliefs
3. Stereotype
4. Ethnonursing

Part 5

1. D
2. C
3. B
4. E
5. A

Part 6

1. B
2. A
3. C
4. B

CHAPTER 9

Part 1

1. 5
2. 1
3. 6
4. 2
5. 4
6. 3

Part 2

1. Complex
2. Any two of the following: transitional, expanding family, contracting family
3. Ethnicity, religion

Part 3

Terms and definitions will vary based on student.

Part 4

1. Extended family
2. Binuclear family
3. Single-parent family
4. Nuclear family

Part 5

1. T
2. F
3. F
4. T
5. F

Part 6

1. E
2. F
3. B
4. A
5. C
6. D

Part 7

1. Any three of the following: socioeconomic stressors, divorce and remarriage, family violence, addictions, acute or chronic illness, or ineffective coping strategies
2. Any two of the following: gay or lesbian family, communal family, foster family

Part 8

1. E
2. E
3. I
4. E
5. I

CHAPTER 10

Part 1

1. Play, anticipatory guidance
2. Newborn
3. Infancy: 1 to 12 months
4. Toddlerhood: 1 to 3 years
5. Preschool: 3 to 6 years
6. School age: 6 to 10 years

Part 2

1. F
2. T
3. T

Part 3

1. C
2. E
3. H
4. B
5. G
6. J
7. A
8. D
9. I
10. F

Part 4

1. Object permanence
2. Interdependent
3. Cephalocaudal

Part 5

1. Tasks
2. 6
3. Nursing bottle mouth is a dental condition with erosion of the tooth enamel, deep cavities, and tooth loss resulting from prolonged contact with milk and juice sugars such as occurs when bottle is propped on a blanket or a towel; can affect appearance, chewing, eating, and speech.

4. Limit setting
5. Preschool

Part 6

1. 2nd, 3rd, 1st, 4th
2. 4th, 2nd, 1st, 3rd
3. Responsibility

CHAPTER 11

Part 1

1. Growth, development, theories
2. Cognitive, emotional, moral
3. Puberty
4. Variation

Part 2

1. C
2. A
3. E
4. B
5. D

Part 3

1. H
2. E
3. P
4. P
5. H

Part 4

1. C
2. B
3. C
4. A

CHAPTER 12

Part 1

1. 3
2. 1
3. 2

Part 2

1. Stability, transition
2. 20, 30; 30, 40
3. Developmental tasks

Part 3

1. Generativity
2. Intimacy
3. Isolation
4. Midlife transition

Part 4

1. M
2. M
3. E
4. M
5. E
6. E
7. M
8. M

Part 5

1. C
2. B
3. E
4. A
5. D

Part 6

1. Choices, circumstances
2. Any three of the following (see text for details).

Leaving the home of origin: can have many patterns including remaining in or near the home.

Choosing a career: occupational choices are closely tied to education and circumstances may affect the individual's adaptability in making adjustments in career dreams; family and friend support is important.

Establishing an adult identification: seeking oneself, seeking to establish roots; individual feels choices can no longer be changed and may fear career or relationship commitment.

Establishing adult relationships: individual forms new friendships and intimate relationships that provide support and understanding after leaving college and the families of origin.

Starting a family: many adults postpone childbirth until their thirties; however, more teenage girls are becoming pregnant. Many couples share child-care responsibilities.

Reappraising commitments: adults may find themselves questioning choices; career and marital changes are considered.

3. Any three of the following: settling in, making career decisions, addressing women's issues, and facing transitions
4. Adjusting to midlife transitions, role changes, mortality, equilibrium, retirement

CHAPTER 13

Part 1

1. Havighurst, Erikson, Levinson, Sheehy
2. Demographics, population trends
3. Continuation
4. Stress, loss, poverty
5. Healthcare

Part 2

1. Mortality—C
2. Ageism—A
3. Gerontology—B

Part 3

1. E
2. H
3. H

4. S
5. E
6. L
7. L
8. E

Part 4

1. I
2. A
3. I
4. I
5. I
6. A
7. A
8. I

Part 5

1. Fixed income
2. Difficulty
3. Volunteerism
4. Connected, same
5. Increase

CHAPTER 14

Part 1

1. 1
2. 4
3. 2
4. 3

Part 2

1. Normal
2. Stress, express, emotions
3. Stages, acceptance

Part 3

1. Reactive depression
2. Detachment

3. Terminal illness
4. Preparatory depression

Part 4

1. T
2. F
3. F
4. F
5. T

Part 5

1. E, J
2. D, L
3. F, K
4. C, G
5. A, H
6. B, I

Part 6

1. Levels:
   1. Drawing strength from God
   2. Strength generated by prayer
   3. Strength from caring relationships with others
2. In some cultures death is a social event with meaning for the entire society, whereas in others death is a private, hidden occurrence; some cultures celebrate the person moving on to a better place, whereas others mourn for extended time; some mourn privately whereas others grieve openly.
3. Anger—rage
   Denial—shock followed by a feeling of isolation
   Bargaining—guilt
   Depression—grief
   Acceptance—self-reliance
   Detachment—decathexis

CHAPTER 15

Part 1

1. A
2. B
3. C
4. A
5. B

Part 2

ATOM

CELL

GENE

CILIA

ORGAN

PLANE

DORSAL

ENZYME

EPONYM

SYSTEM

TISSUE

ACRONYM

ANATOMY

ELEMENT

FRONTAL

MEIOSIS

VENTRAL

MIXTURE

MITOSIS

NUCLEUS

COMPOUND

MEMBRANE

QUADRANT

SAGITTAL

CYTOPLASM

DIAPHRAGM

TRANSVERSE

CHROMOSOME

PROTOPLASM

PHYSIOLOGY

METABOLISM

HOMEOSTASIS

Part 3

1. Space, mixture, kinds, liquid, states
2. Homeostasis, anatomy

Part 4

1. True
2. False Epithelial
3. True
4. False Chemical properties remain unchanged
5. False Not all medical terms have a prefix
6. True

Part 5

1. 111
2. 1,000
3. 2 hydrogen 1 oxygen
4. 99
5. 20
6. 60
7. 3 kinds of matter in 3 states

Part 6

Blood	2
Neurons	4
Calluses	1
Bone	2
Cardiac	3
Glands	1
Adipose	2
Skeletal	3

Part 7

CHAPTER 16

Part 1

1. Skin
2. Accessory structures
3. Thermoregulation
4. Sensory awareness

Part 2

1. Freckles
2. Dermis or true skin
3. Covering
4. Diaphoresis
5. Mammary
6. Thermoregulation

Part 3

1. True
2. False Freckles are patches of melanin clustered together
3. True
4. False White hair results with total loss
5. False Decrease in skin turgor

Part 4

1. Mitotic
2. Protein, dry
3. Evaporation
4. Collagen
5. Subcutaneous

Part 5

1. C
2. B
3. A
4. D
5. C

Part 6

4

CHAPTER 17

Part 1

3, 6, 4, 2, 5, 1

Part 2

Hypertonic	Hypotonic
Acid	Base
Anion	Cation
Extracellular	Intracellular

Part 3

Osmosis	Diffusion
Electrolyte	Ion
Isotonic	Homeostasis
Solute	Salt
Edema	Interstitial

Part 4

1. Inside
2. Positive feedback
3. Homeostasis
4. Anasarca
5. Passive transport
6. Permeability

Part 5

1. C
2. D
3. D

CHAPTER 18

Part 1

1, 5, 3, 4, 2

Part 2

1. G	9. E
2. N	10. O
3. L	11. D
4. M	12. B
5. K	13. H
6. A	14. F
7. C	15. I
8. J	

Part 3

1. Masseter	Structure
2. Joints	Structure
3. Osteoclasts	Function
4. Xiphoid process	Function
5. ATP	Function
6. Manubrium	Structure
7. Acetabulum	Structure
8. Hormones	Function

Part 4

1. "Because of posture and balance adjustments necessary to compensate for the skeletal framework changes, older adults are more likely to fall." (page 197)
2. See Box 18-2 on page 191 for complete listing. Any one from each category is acceptable.

Part 5

1. 25
2. 40
3. 1,000
4. 90,90
5. 28
6. 12

Part 6

Strabismus—cross-eyed

Kyphosis—hunchback

Torticollis—head permanently drawn to one side

Part 7

1. B
2. A
3. D

Part 8

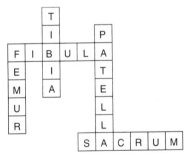

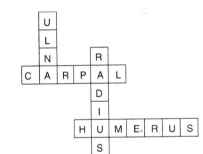

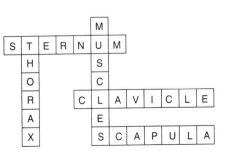

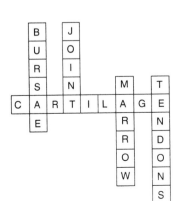

CHAPTER 19

Part 1

1. Cells nervous
2. Central nervous
3. Peripheral nervous
4. Reflexes

Part 2

1. Reflex arc
2. Interneuron
3. Parietal lobe
4. Neurotransmitter
5. Corpus callosum
6. Action potential
7. Hippocampus
8. Reflex
9. Cerebrospinal fluid
10. Decussation
11. Receptors
12. Myelin sheath
13. Neuroglia
14. Cerebellum
15. ANS

Part 3

Sensory	Afferent
Cranial nerve VII	Optic
Parasympathetic	Homeostasis
Cranial nerve II	Facial
Motor	Efferent
Study of nervous system	Neurology
Cranial nerve X	Vagus
Sympathetic	Emergency
Plexus	Group of spinal nerves
Brain and spinal cord	CNS
Neurotransmitter	Acetylcholine
Pons	Bridge

Part 4

1. Mood

2. Arachnoid
3. Dendrite
4. Cerebellum
5. Medulla
6. Communication
7. Occipital
8. Hypothalamus
9. Brain

Part 5

1. Cell
2. From
3. Opposite
4. Milliseconds
5. Involuntary
6. Cannot
7. Frontal
8. Cannot
9. Outermost
10. Pia

CHAPTER 20

Part 1

1. Thyroid
2. Parathyroids
3. Pineal
4. System relationships
5. Negative feedback

Part 2

1. B
2. C
3. D
4. B
5. A

Part 3

A. 4
B. 3
C. 1

D. 2
E. 4
F. 1
G. 2
H. 3
I. 4

Part 4

1. Pituitary
2. Thyroid
3. Pineal
4. Adrenal
5. Pancreas

Part 5

1. True
2. False Fatty acids not hormones
3. True
4. True
5. False Kidney of adults

Part 6

1. Glucagon
2. Pineal gland
3. Adenohypophysis
4. Thymus
5. Pituitary
6. Thyroid
7. Adrenals
8. Glycogen

Part 7

1. T
2. F Essential
3. F Endocrine
4. F Fatty acids
5. T
6. T
7. F Tiny
8. T
9. T
10. F Blood transports hormones

CHAPTER 21

Part 1

1. A
2. B
3. B
4. C
5. B

Part 2

1. Cerumen
2. Accommodation
3. Lacrimal glands
4. Ossicles
5. Vitreous humor
6. Cochlea
7. Proprioceptors
8. Rods
9. Myopia
10. Optic disk

Part 3

1. Sight—eye, hearing—ear, taste—tongue, smell—nose, touch—skin
2. Cranial nerves II—optic, III—ocular motor
3. Inner ear, semicircular canal
4. See page 228: any three of those listed in Table 21-1: superior, inferior, lateral, and medial rectus, and superior or inferior oblique
5. Middle ear

Part 4

1. Presbyopia
2. Presbycusis

Part 5

1. Chemoreceptors
2. Rods
3. Occipital

4. Opens
5. Cranial nerve III oculomotor; cranial nerve I olfactory

Part 6

1. B
2. C
3. A
4. D

CHAPTER 22

Part 1

1. System physiology
2. Cardiac conduction
3. Aging . . . system
4. Blood vessels
5. Cardiac output

Part 2

1. G
2. I
3. H
4. J
5. B
6. F
7. C
8. A
9. D
10. E

Part 3

1. **Myo**cardium
2. **Endo**cardium
3. **Epi**cardium
4. **Peri**cardium
5. **Semilunar** valves
6. **Tricuspid** valve

7. **AV** valves
8. **Mitral (or bicuspid)** valve

Part 4

1. They fit over the heart like a crown (corona).
2. Because of the crescent or half-moon shape of its cusps
3. Ventricles filling creates audible vibrations during a time of diastole that would normally be a silent phase of the heart.

Part 5

1. Unidirectional
2. Normal
3. Right
4. Septum
5. Mediastinum
6. SA
7. Systole
8. Capillaries
9. Apex
10. Papillary

Part 6

1. (Result of aging) Any two of the following (see page 245 for details): number of pacemaker cells decrease in the SA node, decrease in fibers in bundle of His, and increase in ectopic heart beats
2. Tricuspid valve between right atria and right ventricle. Bicuspid or mitral between the left atria and left ventricle.
3. For details see page 244—the greater the stretch the greater the force of contraction.
4. The autonomic nerves send input from cardiac center in the medulla to the heart (see page 242).

Part 7

Explain what blood pressure is and factors that influence it (see page 244).

Part 8

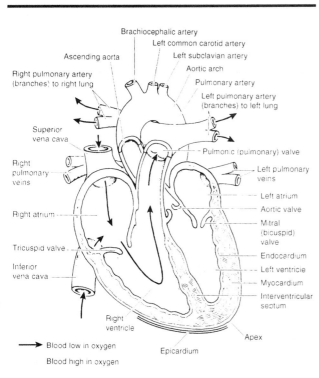

Brachiocephalic artery
Left common carotid artery
Ascending aorta
Left subclavian artery
Aortic arch
Right pulmonary artery
(branches) to right lung
Pulmonary artery
Left pulmonary artery
(branches) to left lung
Superior
vena cava
Pulmonic (pulmonary) valve
Right
pulmonary
veins
Left pulmonary
veins
Left atrium
Aortic valve
Right atrium
Mitral
(bicuspid)
valve
Tricuspid valve
Endocardium
Left ventricle
Inferior
vena cava
Myocardium
Interventricular
septum
Right
ventricle
Apex
→ Blood low in oxygen
Epicardium
Blood high in oxygen

CHAPTER 23

Part 1

1. B
2. A
3. A
4. B

Part 2

1. K
2. F
3. B
4. I
5. M
6. L
7. O
8. C
9. E
10. A
11. N
12. H
13. D

14. G
15. J

Part 3

1. D
2. B
3. B
4. C
5. A

Part 4

1. True
2. True
3. False Watery
4. False 90%
5. True
6. False Incompatible
7. True
8. False Small intestine
9. True
10. False Inferior vena cava
11. True
12. True
13. True
14. False Capillaries
15. True

Part 5

1. 55
2. 120
3. 25
4. 4
5. 3
6. 1
7. 45
8. 10
9. 6
10. 80

Part 6

1. Lymph nodes may function to filter out cancer cells or may inadvertently spread cancer to other body sites (see page 252 for details).
2. If cancer is found in the lymph nodes it is said to be spreading or metastasized.

CHAPTER 24

Part 1

5

1

3

2

4

Part 2

1. C
2. B
3. A
4. B
5. C

Part 3

1. B cells
2. Don't
3. T cells
4. Humeral
5. Rejection
6. Primary
7. Lungs
8. Stimulates
9. Antigens
10. Atrophy

Part 4

1. Interferon
2. Immunoglobulins
3. B
4. Defense
5. Overreactive

Part 5

1. After birth, the baby can receive protection through the mother's breast milk. This protection lasts up to 6 months, when the infant's own immune system begins to take over (see page 260).

CHAPTER 25

Part 1

1. Upper respiratory tract, gas exchange
2. Effects of aging on the system

Part 2

1. C   Effects of aging
2. A   System physiology
3. A   System physiology
4. B   Structure and function
5. C   System physiology

Part 3

1. External respiration
2. Intercostal muscles
3. Tidal volume
4. Cellular or internal respiration
5. Vital capacity

Part 4

1. False Trachea and esophagus are located in the pharynx.
2. False Pleura has two layers.
3. True
4. False External respiration is exchange of gas at lung level *or* Internal respiration is exchange of gas at the cellular level.
5. True

Part 5

1. Diaphragm
2. Larynx
3. Alveolar ducts
4. Hilum
5. Oropharynx
6. Pleural cavity
7. Laryngopharynx
8. Apex
9. Medulla
10. Epiglottis

CHAPTER 26

Part 1

1. Not sterile
2. Duodenum
3. Liver
4. Small
5. Vitamin K and B complex

Part 2

1. G
2. H
3. J
4. F
5. B

6. I
7. D
8. E
9. A
10. C

Part 3

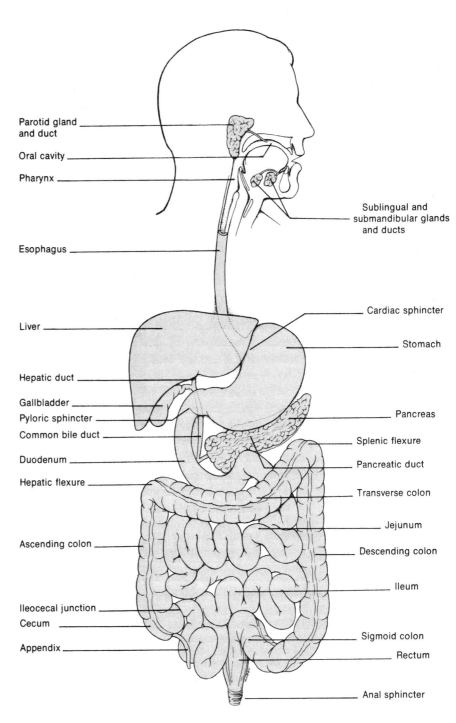

Parotid gland and duct
Oral cavity
Pharynx
Sublingual and submandibular glands and ducts
Esophagus
Cardiac sphincter
Liver
Stomach
Hepatic duct
Gallbladder
Pyloric sphincter
Common bile duct
Pancreas
Duodenum
Splenic flexure
Pancreatic duct
Hepatic flexure
Transverse colon
Jejunum
Ascending colon
Descending colon
Ileum
Ileocecal junction
Cecum
Sigmoid colon
Appendix
Rectum
Anal sphincter

Part 4

1. B
2. D
3. D
4. C
5. A

Part 5

1. 8
2. 1
3. 4
4. 5
5. 2

CHAPTER 27

Part 1

1. Ureters
2. Urine formation and micturition
3. Wastes, volume, electrolyte, pH, D, renin, and erythropoietin

Part 2

1. False Forming not expelling urine
2. True
3. False Stores not forms
4. True
5. False 95%
6. False Posterior (behind)
7. True
8. False Renal medulla
9. False 10%
10. False Formation of urine

Part 3

1. Micturition
2. Retroperitoneal
3. Nephron
4. Renin
5. Edema
6. Pinocytosis
7. Nocturia
8. Ureters
9. Erythropoietin
10. Water

Part 4

Note color, clarity, and odor.

Urine is initially a clear, amber liquid with a characteristic odor.

Abnormal products include blood, pus, casts.

See page 288.

CHAPTER 28

Part 1

1. C
2. B
3. B
4. A
5. D
6. B

Part 2

1. Testosterone
2. Prostate
3. Copulation
4. Testes
5. Circumcision

Part 3

1. False Men do not normally stop producing sperm.
2. False Located inferior (below) the prostate
3. True
4. True
5. True

CHAPTER 29

Part 1

1. Oviducts   Structure
2. Changes associated with aging   Effects of aging
3. Menstrual cycle   Physiology
4. Breasts   Structure
5. Sexual response   Physiology

Part 2

1. Mons pubis
2. Progesterone
3. Bartholin's glands
4. Oocyte
5. Gonadotrophin hormone

Part 3

1. 16
2. 28
3. 2
4. 14
5. 3

Part 4

1. Oocyte
2. Menopause
3. Estrogens
4. After
5. Fallopian tube
6. External
7. Anus
8. Endometrium
9. Luteal
10. Fundus

Part 5

Ovary	Gonad
Painful intercourse	Dyspareunia
Zygote	Fertilized ovum
Oviduct	Fallopian tube
Mature oocyte	Ovum
Uterus	Womb
Clitoris	Penis

CHAPTER 30

Part 1

1. N
2. HD

3. NAL
4. NAL
5. N

Part 2

1. Recommended Dietary Allowances
2. Empty calories
3. Essential nutrients
4. Nutrient density
5. Body mass index
6. Resting energy expenditure
7. Enzyme
8. Kilocalorie
9. Energy
10. Malnutrition

Part 3

1. C, F
2. A, D
3. B, E

Part 4

1. Preventing, reducing, risk
2. Water, minerals, and vitamins
3. Water, thirst
4. Minerals
5. Vitamins
6. Overweight, obese

Part 5

1. I
2. I
3. A
4. A
5. I
6. A
7. A
8. I

Part 6

1. F
2. T
3. T

4. F
5. T

Part 7

1. B—130 lb
2. A—28
3. D—Overnutrition contributes to such conditions as hypertension and osteoporosis.
4. C—Not worry, as long as Niketa has reasonable intake from each of the major food groups

Part 8

1. Fruits—C
2. Vegetables—B
3. Meat—E
4. Milk—D
5. Grain—A
6. Other—F

CHAPTER 31

Part I

1. Vegetarian—Choice
2. Religious—Beliefs
3. Regional—Preferences
4. Ethnic—Heritage

Part 2

1. Transcultural
2. Ethnic, religious
3. B_{12}, D

Part 3

1. Kosher
2. Tofu
3. Soul food
4. Lacto-ovo

Part 4

1. I   6. I
2. I   7. A
3. A   8. A
4. I   9. A
5. A   10. A

Part 5

1. C
2. A
3. B
4. E
5. C

CHAPTER 32

Part 1

1. 2
2. 5
3. 1
4. 3
5. 6
6. 4

Part 2

1. T
2. F
3. T
4. T

Part 3

1. Low-residue
2. Fat-controlled, elevated
3. Are not
4. Low
5. Carbohydrate-controlled diet
6. Total parenteral nutrition (TPN)

Part 4

1. Dysphagia
2. Hyperlipidemia
3. Anorexia
4. Edema
5. Peripheral parenteral nutrition (PPN)

Part 5

1. C
2. D
3. A
4. E
5. B

Part 6

1. 3
2. 5
3. 2
4. 6
5. 4
6. 1

CHAPTER 33

Part 1

1. 5
2. 1
3. 4
4. 2
5. 3

Part 2

1. T
2. F
3. F
4. T

Part 3

1. Trial and error

2. Critical thinking
3. Nursing process
4. Client-oriented
5. Nursing care plans

Part 4

1. Planning
2. Evaluation
3. Assessment
4. Implementation
5. Diagnosis

Part 5

1. C
2. E
3. A
4. B
5. D

Part 6

Critical thinking is a method of problem-solving that is neither trial and error nor structured scientific problem-solving system; it uses a complicated mix of inquiry, knowledge, intuition, logic, experience, and common sense.

CHAPTER 34

Part 1

1. B
2. A
3. B
4. B
5. A

Part 2

1. Objective data
2. Health interview
3. Observation
4. Subjective data
5. Data analysis

Part 3

1. B
2. C
3. A
4. B
5. C

Part 4

1. Recognizing significant data—involves asking yourself which data items are pertinent to client care
   Validating observations—involves determining if your observations agree with what the client is experiencing; you also may consult colleagues or the nursing team leader
   Recognizing patterns or clusters—involves noting what data are similar or have a pattern or connection
   Identifying strengths and analyzing problems—includes looking for coping skills the client has for handling problems and noting which problems are actual and which are potential
   Reaching conclusions—determining if the client has no problem, may have a problem but additional information is needed, is at risk for a problem, or has a clinical problem with a nursing diagnosis or medical diagnosis
2. Collection, analysis
3. Client, family

Part 5

1. D
2. B

CHAPTER 35

Part 1

1. B
2. B
3. A
4. A
5. B

Part 2

1. Expected outcome

2. Medical diagnosis
3. Nursing diagnosis
4. Kardex
5. Collaborative problem

Part 3

1. N
2. M
3. N
4. N
5. M

Part 4

1. Problem, etiology, signs and symptoms
2. In *setting priorities*, the nurse considers all nursing diagnoses to determine which are most important and which are less important. *Establishing expected outcomes* involves the nurse working with the client and family to establish measurable client goals or objectives that are client oriented, specific, reasonable, and measurable. In *selecting nursing interventions*, the nurse determines activities that will most likely produce the desired outcomes. In writing a nursing care plan the nursing team, in a nursing care conference, writes a formal guideline for directing nursing staff, which usually includes nursing diagnoses or client problems, expected outcomes, and nursing orders.

Part 5

1. S
2. P
3. T
4. T
5. T
6. P

CHAPTER 36

Part 1

1. B
2. A
3. C
4. B

5. A
6. C

Part 2

1. Implementation
2. Dependent actions
3. Accountability
4. Interpersonal skills
5. Intellectual skills
6. Quality assurance
7. Chart audit
8. Nursing peer review

Part 3

1. D
2. G
3. F
4. H
5. C
6. A
7. E
8. B

Part 4

1. Communicating, documenting
2. Analyzing the client's responses, identifying factors contributing to success or failure, and planning for future care

Part 5

1. C
2. B
3. D

CHAPTER 37

Part 1

1. 3
2. 5
3. 2

4. 1
5. 4

Part 2

1. Timely, precise
2. Manual and electronic
3. Confidentiality
4. Record, client

Part 3

1. Health record
2. Medical information
3. Flow sheet
4. Minimum data set
5. Resident assessment
6. Progress note

Part 4

1. Communication, accountability, health research, education
2. Walking rounds
3. Change-of-shift
4. Manual, electronic
5. Assessment, care, treatment, progress, continuity, care

Part 5

1. A
2. I
3. I
4. A
5. A
6. I
7. I
8. A

Part 6

1. D
2. F
3. I
4. A
5. E

6. B
7. C
8. J
9. G
10. H

CHAPTER 38

Part 1

1. CU
2. HP
3. CU
4. HP
5. HP

Part 2

1. Client unit
2. Clinics, home
3. Clean, orderly
4. Mayo stand
5. Morgue

Part 3

1. E
2. F
3. G
4. D
5. C
6. H
7. B
8. A

Part 4

1. Coronary care unit
2. Pediatric
3. Rehabilitation unit
4. Emergency department
5. Obstetrics
6. Hospice
7. Central service supply
8. Quality improvement department
9. Housekeeping
10. Chemical dependency unit

Part 5

1. Standard
2. Your hands
3. Hurt, painful
4. Comfortable
5. Examinations
6. Help

CHAPTER 39

Part 1

1. FP
2. S&P
3. DP
4. FP
5. S&P

Part 2

1. Hazardous
2. Knowledgeable
3. Prevent, what to do

Part 3

1. Triage
2. Disaster medical assistance
3. Simple, rapid treatment
4. External
5. Command center
6. Internal
7. Rescue, alert/alarm, confine, extinguish
8. Disaster plan

Part 4

1. Any five of the following:

   Read labels carefully and note emergency information.

   Follow instructions for use, storage, and disposal.

   Avoid spills.

   Use protective equipment as recommended.

   Do not store hazardous materials in familiar food or drink containers.

Keep household chemicals in their original containers.

Do not use gasoline indoors.
2. Poisons, skin/eye irritants, carcinogens.
3. A—Obstacles
   B—Tangles loose plugs fraying
   C—Assistance
   D—Side rails
   E—Lighting

Part 5

1. A
2. B, C
3. B, C
4. A, B, C

CHAPTER 40

Part 1

1. A
2. B
3. A
4. C
5. B

Part 2

1. Communicable
2. Contagious
3. Mycosis
4. Vector
5. Exotoxins
6. Parasites
7. Suppurative
8. Toxin
9. Pathogen
10. Virulence

Part 3

1. D
2. E
3. C
4. A
5. F
6. B

Part 4

1. Portal, entry, microorganisms, virulence, resistance
2. Algae: resemble plant cells, rarely cause human disease

   Fungi: include yeasts and molds (common in the environment), cause ringworm

   Protozoa: single-celled, live in moisture-rich environment; ameba and paramecium; although most are nonpathogenic, malaria, dysentery, and *Trichomonas vaginalis* infection may result from some types.

   Bacteria: single-celled organism without a true nucleus, DNA floats freely within cytoplasm; may be gram positive or negative, aerobic or anaerobic, may become resistant.

   Viruses are protein-covered sacs containing either DNA or RNA; they use the host cell of a living organism to produce protein and energy and to replicate.
3. Take antibiotics only as prescribed.

   Take antibiotics for the entire period prescribed.

   Do not share antibiotics with others or take their "leftover medication."

   Discuss the necessity of antibiotics for mild bacterial infections with your healthcare provider.

Part 5

1. A
2. D
3. B
4. C
5. E

CHAPTER 41

Part 1

1. 5
2. 1
3. 2
4. 4
5. 3

Part 2

1. Nosocomial
2. Gloves, gowns, masks

3. Aseptic
4. Medical asepsis

Part 3

1. Personal protective equipment
2. Medical asepsis
3. Antimicrobial agents
4. Invasive
5. Endogenous
6. Bacteremias

Part 4

1. Handwashing; barrier; clean, controlled
2. 10–15, longer
3. Any three of the following: broad-spectrum antibiotics are used frequently, healthcare personnel fail to use appropriate proper techniques, multiple healthcare personnel provide care for a client, the client experiences a prolonged hospitalization, or a person has a lowered resistance to disease.
4. Mask, eye, gloves
5. Number, kinds; exit and entry; spread, site to grow

Part 5

1. I
2. A
3. I
4. A
5. A
6. I
7. A
8. I

CHAPTER 42

Part 1

1. Control
2. Respirator masks
3. Protective
4. Barrier
5. Control committee

Part 2

1. D
2. E
3. B
4. A
5. C

Part 3

1. Colonization
2. Sweat, skin, mucous
3. Contact
4. Mask, eye protection, face shield
5. Handwashing, gloves
6. Handwashing, gloves, gown, mask, eyewear
7. Stand, PPE
8. Disposable, disposable

Part 4

1. M, H
2. H, Gl
3. H, Gl, M, G, E
4. N
5. M, MC, Gl

CHAPTER 43

Part 1

1. Sudden death and life support
2. Progress, is not, progress
3. Standard Precautions
4. 911
5. Shock

Part 2

Responses will vary with student choices of terms, definitions in text.

Part 3

1. E
2. H

3. I
4. F
5. J
6. A
7. D
8. C
9. B
10. G

Part 4

1. A
2. A
3. I
4. A
5. I
6. A
7. A
8. A
9. I
10. I

Part 5

1. Clinical, biologic, biologic
2. Sudden
3. Automated external defibrillator
4. Breathing, circulation, disability, exposure and examine
5. Exhaustion, stroke
6. Rest, ice, compression, elevation

Part 6

1. 4
2. 8
3. 3
4. 5
5. 2
6. 6
7. 1
8. 7

CHAPTER 44

Part 1

1. A
2. C

3. B
4. B
5. A

Part 2

1. False Goal directed
2. True
3. False Inability
4. True
5. True

Part 3

Students cannot take verbal orders (see page 483 of text).

Part 4

1. Any two of the nine factors listed in Table: "Factors affecting communication" (see page 480 of text).
2. Barriers
3. Eye contact
4. Protocols
5. Message, receiver

CHAPTER 45

Part 1

3

1

4

2

Part 2

1. C
2. B
3. B
4. C
5. D
6. A

Part 3

1. Transfer
2. Discharge
3. Discharge
4. Transfer
5. Admission

Part 4

1. No liability
2. Daily
3. Regression
4. Anxiety
5. Identification band
6. Dehumanization

CHAPTER 46

Part 1

1. Graphic record
2. Equipment, pulse, respiration, blood pressure
3. Collect information, well-being
4. Pulse
5. Respiration

Part 2

1. C
2. A
3. D
4. B
5. D

Part 3

1. No. Normal blood pressure reading 120/80
2. 130
3. Oral, easiest, least invasive, most comfortable (see page 501 of the text)
4. Terms such as regular, irregular, or weak could be used (see page 506 of the text).
5. Eupnea

Part 4

1. False Cannot be used interchangeably
2. True
3. False Accidental hypothermia
4. True
5. True

CHAPTER 47

Part 1

1. Factors, influence, assessment
2. Laboratory tests
3. Disease, illness
4. Etiology, effect
5. Head-to-toe, body systems

Part 2

1. G
2. D
3. E
4. H
5. F
6. I
7. B
8. J
9. C
10. A

Part 3

1. Pulse oximetry
2. Palpation
3. Biopsy
4. Correct as is: cardiac catheterization
5. Endoscopy
6. Inspection
7. Electrocardiogram
8. MRI or CT scan

Part 4

1. D
2. A
3. D
4. B

CHAPTER 48

Part 1

1. Positioning, examinations
2. Safety, paralyzed
3. Pulling, rolling, start, stop
4. Dizzy

Part 2

1. J
2. D
3. H
4. A
5. B
6. E
7. G
8. I
9. C
10. F

Part 3

1. A
2. I
3. A
4. I
5. I
6. A

Part 4

1. Any three of the following: (1) It is easier to pull, push, or roll an object than it is to lift it, the movement should be smooth and continuous rather than jerky; (2) often less energy or force is required to keep an object moving than it is to start and stop it; (3) it takes less effort to lift an object if you work as close to it as possible. Use your leg and arm muscles as much as possible and your back muscles, which are not as strong as little as possible. Avoid reaching; or (4) rocking backward or forward on your feet uses your body weight as a force for pulling or pushing.
2. Wide
3. Pelvic
4. Alignment
5. Gravital

Part 5

1. 5
2. 3
3. 1
4. 7
5. 8
6. 6
7. 2
8. 4

CHAPTER 49

Part 1

1. Special, mattresses
2. Cradle, rails, equipment
3. Work, before, one, time, energy
4. Soiled, chair

Part 2

1. C
2. D
3. A
4. B
5. E

Part 3

1. A
2. I
3. A
4. I
5. I
6. A

Part 4

1. P
2. O
3. C

Part 5

1. 4
2. 2
3. 5
4. 1
5. 3
6. 6

Part 6

1. Prevent, assistive
2. Any two of the following: clients with fractures, extensive burns, or open or painful wounds
3. Support, correct alignment
4. Contractures, immobility, wounds
5. Pressure

CHAPTER 50

Part 1

1. Routine eye care, ear care
2. Fingernails, toenails, shaving
3. Much, self-care
4. Backrub, skin

Part 2

1. D
2. E
3. C
4. B
5. A

Part 3

1. A
2. A
3. I
4. A
5. A
6. I
7. I
8. A

9. I
10. I

Part 4

1. Any three of the following, see book for additional details. Many disease-causing organisms enter the body through the mouth; food particles between teeth cause complications; some illnesses cause sores to develop; some gum infections are transmitted from person to person; a mouth condition may decrease appetite; oral conditions may cause pain or infection in other body parts; and breath odors or decaying teeth make people self-conscious.
2. Towel bath may be given when water should not be used on the client, a partial bed bath may be given on days when a complete bath is omitted or the client is able to do part of the bath, and the complete bath is given when client cannot move and requires complete assistance.
3. Straight across
4. Unsteady, eyesight
5. Front

Part 5

1. 6
2. 3
3. 4
4. 1
5. 8
6. 11
7. 2
8. 12
9. 7
10. 5
11. 9
12. 10

CHAPTER 51

Part 1

1. C
2. D
3. D
4. A
5. B
6. C

Part 2

1. Diarrhea
2. Comfortable, privacy
3. Elimination, life

Part 3

1. Defecation
2. Oliguria
3. Nocturia
4. Dysuria
5. Retention
6. Anuria

Part 4

1. C
2. A
3. G
4. F
5. H
6. B
7. D
8. E

Part 5

1. Freshly voided urine is generally light yellow or amber, clear, has an aromatic odor, is 250 to 400 mL and contains no abnormal components such as blood or pus.
2. Micturition, voiding.
3. Appearance: the presence of pus or mucus may indicate inflammation or infection; undigested food may indicate digestive system malfunction, blood may indicate hemorrhage; color changes may indicate missing bile (clay color), bleeding (black), or yellow (microorganisms); consistency changes may occur with stress (diarrhea or constipation); in addition, constipation may occur if client is dehydrated and diarrhea may occur if client has chronic irritation or a parasitic infection; odor changes may occur with the presence of microorganisms or the ingestion of some medications.
4. Feces
5. Any three of the following: cleansing enema is given to stimulate peristalsis, soften feces, and produce a bowel movement to empty the rectum and lower colon; carminative enema is given to stimulate peristalsis and the expelling of flatus, an anthelmininthic drug may be given as a retention enema to kill parasites; emollient enema may be given to protect or soothe the mucous membranes; oil enema is given to stimulate bowel evacuation; medicated enema may be given to administer a drug because the drug may be rapidly absorbed by the colon's mucous membranes.

Part 6

1. 8
2. 3
3. 6
4. 9
5. 5
6. 10
7. 4
8. 1
9. 7
10. 2

CHAPTER 52

Part 1

3rd

2nd

4th

1st

Part 2

1. Education, practice
2. Abnormal
3. Precautions
4. Early, morning

Part 3

1. Expectorate
2. Hydrometer
3. Urinalysis
4. Specific gravity
5. Hemoccult
6. Venipuncture

Part 4

1. T
2. F
3. F
4. F
5. T
6. F

Part 5

1. G
2. J
3. A

4. C
5. B

Part 6

1. Clamp, collection
2. Discard
3. Awakens
4. Wear, gloves
5. Three

CHAPTER 53

Part 1

Ba

Bi

Ba

Part 2

1. Antiembolism stocking
2. Binders
3. Body parts

Part 3

1. C
2. E
3. D

4. A
5. B

Part 4

1. Elasticized, support, dressings
2. Around
3. Firmly, tightly
4. Shave
5. Gloves, waist, perineal, between, midline

CHAPTER 54

Part 1

1. *Rules* for *application*
2. Heat, cold
3. *Dilates*
4. *Sitz bath*
5. *Small*

Part 2

1. C
2. A
3. E
4. D
5. B

Part 3

1. C
2. C
3. H
4. H
5. C
6. C
7. H
8. C

Part 4

1. Slowing, congestion
2. Change
3. ¾
4. Clean gloves
5. Petroleum jelly
6. Insulate against heat loss and moisture evaporation
7. Breathing
8. Axillae, groin

Part 5

1. I
2. I
3. A

4. A
5. I

CHAPTER 55

Part 1

1. Nursing assessment
2. Chronic/neuropathic
3. Early
4. Surgical intervention
5. Transduction, transmission, perception, modulation
6. Location, duration, quantity, quality, aggravating/alleviating factors, and related occurrences

Part 2

1. C
2. H
3. E
4. A
5. F
6. D
7. G
8. B

Part 3

1. Nociception
2. Distraction and diversion
3. Stress
4. Nonsteroidal anti-inflammatory drugs (NSAIDs), mild to moderate, opioids/narcotic analgesics, severe, adjuvant drugs, mood
5. Surgery

Part 4

1. I
2. A
3. A
4. A
5. I
6. I

Part 5

1. A
2. D
3. B
4. C

CHAPTER 56

Part 1

1. B
2. B
3. A
4. D
5. A
6. D

Part 2

1. Intraoperative
2. Teaching
3. Hypoxia, hypothermia
4. Pulmonary

Part 3

1. H
2. J
3. G
4. F
5. C
6. A
7. B
8. I
9. D
10. E

Part 4

1. A
2. I
3. A
4. A
5. I

Part 5

1. B
2. A
3. C
4. D

CHAPTER 57

Part 1

1. 3
2. 1
3. 4
4. 2

Part 2

1. Clean, many
2. Contaminated
3. Sterile procedure
4. Sterile technique

Part 3

1. Surgical asepsis
2. Sterile technique
3. Dirty
4. Autoclave
5. Disinfection

Part 4

1. T	4. F
2. T	5. F
3. F	6. T

Part 5

A. 2, 4, 1, 5, 3

B. 3, 4, 1, 9, 7, 10, 2, 8, 5, 6

CHAPTER 58

Part 1

1. Wounds, skin breakdown
2. First, second, third
3. Eliminating, causes
4. Wound

Part 2

1. H	6. D
2. F	7. J
3. C	8. B
4. G	9. I
5. A	10. E

Part 3

1. F	4. F
2. T	5. T
3. T	6. F

Part 4

1. A	4. I
2. A	5. A
3. I	

Part 5

1. Pressure—bony prominences such as occiput, dorsal thoracic area, elbow, sacrum, heel (see Fig. 58-2 for additional sites)
   Shear—surfaces exposed to bed or chair
   Friction—surfaces that rub on bed or chair surfaces
   Stripping—surfaces where tape applied
   Urine or stool—perianal skin
   Perspiration—areas where moisture can get, such as skin folds
   Arterial insufficiency—feet, toes, lower leg
2. See Table 58-1 for additional measures.
   Pressure—establish and implementing a turning schedule at least every 2 hours
   Shear—use draw sheets, limit elevation of head of bed
   Friction—apply transparent dressings to areas of friction, move client carefully
   Stripping—use only porous tapes and apply without tension
   Urine or stool—use containment equipment such as absorptive products, or condom catheters
   Perspiration—keep areas of skin folds dry, use barrier ointments
   Arterial insufficiency—avoid compression, protect from mechanical, chemical, or hermal injuries

CHAPTER 59

Part 1

1. Coping, dead, person's, body; and coping, client's, death
2. Role, hope
3. Position
4. Ease
5. Physical

Part 2

1. Kussmaul's breathing
2. Apnea
3. Hyperpnea
4. Autopsy
5. Cheyne-Stokes respirations
6. Biologic death

Part 3

1. See pages 141 to 143 of text for more details. Care of the mouth, nose, and eyes: swab the client's mouth with mouthwash to keep it clean, turn the client to promote drainage, free the nostrils of crust, moisten the tongue, wipe eyes with moist cotton balls or gauze; breathing difficulties can be reduced with turning the client onto the side or propping the client up into a partially sitting position; incontinent clients should be kept clean and dry; nutrition may be provided through tube feedings or TPN; odor control involves keeping dressings clean and dry and drainage bags empty as well as managing incontinence and using subtle deodorizers.
2. Failing circulation and failing senses are signs of approaching death.
3. Straighten, top, sheet
   List, sign
   Home, family

Part 4

1. D
2. E
3. C
4. B
5. A

CHAPTER 60

Part 1

1. Household, metric, apothecary
2. Dosage, calculation
3. Convert, drug dosage, unit, measurement
4. Ratios, proportions, fractions, significant figures, percentages

Part 2

1. B
2. A
3. C
4. B
5. C
6. A

Part 3

1. E
2. D
3. A
4. F
5. C

Part 4

1. Because you are converting from a smaller to a larger unit, you would divide milligrams by 1000 (move the decimal to the left).
2. First write the problem, second invert the divisor, then multiply the numerators and denominators.
3. Smaller, half.
4. Double-check the dosage conversions using a reference book or table; have another nurse double-check the calculations.

Part 5

1. C—set up the problem: $(D)/(A) \times$ quantity = $1/100$ divided by $1/200 \times 1$ tablet = $1/100 \times 200/1 = 200/100 = 2$ tablets *or* $1/100$ gr : 1 tab :: $1/200$ gr : $\times$ tab = $1/100 \times :: 1/200 \rightarrow \times = 200/100 = 2$
2. D—30% = $30/100 \times 3,000/1 = 30 \times 3,000/100 = 90,000/100 = 900$
3. B—$(D)/(A) \times$ quantity = 60 mg/120 mg $\times$ 1 mL = 0.5 $\times 5 = 2.5$
4. C—consult the table of equivalents and set up the problem $\rightarrow$ 1 tsp: 5 mL :: 2 tsp: X $\rightarrow$ X = 10 mL
5. A—50 mL : 1 hour :: 250 mL : X $\rightarrow$ 50X : 250 mL $\rightarrow$ X = 250/50 = 5 hours

CHAPTER 61

Part 1

3, 1, 2

Part 2

1. Drug references, websites
2. Names, actions, forms

Part 3

Response will vary with student selection of unknown terms; see textbook for definitions.

Part 4

1. Dosage
2. Transdermal
3. Pharmacology
4. Enteric-coated
5. Caplet

Part 5

1. F
2. T
3. F
4. T
5. T

Part 6

1. E
2. J
3. A
4. I
5. H
6. D
7. F
8. G
9. C
10. B

Part 7

1. Any three of the following would be correct: the drug classification, use, recommended dosage, desired effects, possible adverse or untoward effects, and route of administration.
2. Intramuscular, subcutaneous, intradermal, intravenous
3. Any four of the following would be correct: age, gender, weight, condition, disposition and psychological state, method of administration, distribution, environment, time of administration, or elimination.

CHAPTER 62

Part 1

1. Antineoplastic
2. Integumentary
3. Antibiotics, anti-infective

Part 2

1. Current drug reference
2. Endocrine

Part 3

1. Bactericidal
2. Catecholamine
3. Sedative
4. Hypnotic
5. Cathartic

Part 4

1. C
2. H
3. G
4. I
5. E
6. J
7. A
8. D
9. F
10. B

Part 5

1. Penicillins—inhibit growth of bacteria, allergic reaction, sensitivity, (amoxicillin/Amoxil), bactericidal in high concentrations
2. Hypnotics—produce sedation and sleep; drowsiness, lethargy, depression, (phenobarbital/Luminal), control seizures, addiction, physical dependence
3. NSAIDs—nonsteroidal, treat inflammation, anal-

gesics, gastric upset, anti-inflammatory drugs and antipyretics
4. Adrenergic medications—neurotransmitters play part in epinephrine (Adrenalin), mimic the actions of the sympathetic, nervousness, tachycardia/parasympathetic nervous systems, heart palpitations, nausea, constrict blood vessels; bronchodilation, tremors, severe headache
5. Steroids—effective anti-inflammatory agent, cushingoid side effects, prednisone (Delta-Cortef), thrombophlebitis, adrenal crisis if suddenly discontinued

Part 6

1. Antibiotic-resistant
2. Stimulants, depressants
3. Any five of the following: euphoria, increased appetite and weight gain, tendency to bruise, hirsutism, adolescent acne, weakness, hypertension, high blood glucose, susceptibility to infection, cataract formation, thrombophlebitis/embolism, moon face, buffalo hump, osteoporosis

Part 7

1. C
2. D
3. A
4. B

CHAPTER 63

Part 1

1. B
2. C
3. E
4. A
5. E
6. D

Part 2

1. Adverse
2. Infiltration
3. Transfusion
4. Anaphylactic
5. Toxicity

Part 3

1. Medication administration record
2. Local, systemic
3. Right client, right medication, right dose, right time, and right route
4. Parenteral

Part 4

1. F
2. F
3. T
4. T
5. F

Part 5

1. TPN—total parenteral nutrition, IV—intravenous, PICC—percutaneous intravenous central catheter
2. STAT—immediately, TD—transdermal, S—sublingual
3. IVPB—intravenous (IV) piggyback, DRF—drip rate factor

Part 6

1. B, F
2. D, G
3. E, G
4. A, F
5. C, G

Part 7

1. 3, 6, 4, 1, 5, 2
2. 4, 5, 3, 2, 1
3. 4, 6, 7, 10, 3, 9, 2, 5, 8, 1

CHAPTER 64

Part 1

Mi

Ma

Mi
Mi
Ma
Ma

4. Not harmful
5. First
6. Morning sickness, frequent small, dry
7. Preparation, parenthood
8. Antepartal classes
9. Natural childbirth
10. Expectations, physical, emotional

Part 2

1. Teratogen
2. Antepartal
3. Continue

Part 3

1. A
2. I
3. B
4. D
5. C
6. F
7. E
8. J
9. G
10. H

Part 4

1. T
2. F
3. T
4. T
5. F

Part 5

1. Quickening
2. Hyperemesis gravidarum
3. Pica
4. Ballottement

Part 6

1. 300
2. Softener, fiber, laxatives
3. Soap

CHAPTER 65

Part 1

1. Labor
2. Second
3. Postpartum

Part 2

1. Recognize
2. Delivery, placenta
3. Changes/involution
4. 3, 5

Part 3

1. Lightening
2. Colostrum
3. Dilation
4. Effacement
5. Afterpains
6. Crowning

Part 4

1. C
2. A
3. B
4. A
5. D
6. C
7. C
8. D

Part 5

1. Spontaneous rupture, membranes; artificially rupture, membranes
2. Longitudinal, transverse
3. Latent; active; transitional
4. Any five of the following: sharp, unremitting pain, prolonged contractions or failure of the uterus to relax, change in character of the fetal heartbeat-abnormal deceleration pattern, bleeding, extreme maternal exhaustion, cessation of labor after it has begun, hypotension or increased pulse rate of the mother, prolapse of the umbilical cord, irregular fetal heartbeat, passage of meconium-stained amniotic fluid when fetus is in vertex position, exaggerated movement of the fetus, or a pH value below 7.2 of fetal blood.
5. 0, engaged
6. True Labor
   Regular, rhythmic contractions
   Increase in duration, frequency
   Increase on ambulation
   Start in back, radiate to abdomen
   Cervix dilates and effaces
   "Show" usually present
   False Labor
   Contractions irregular
   Do not increase in duration, frequency, and intensity
   Decrease on ambulation
   Primarily located in lower abdomen
   No cervical changes
   "Show" absent

CHAPTER 66

Part 1

1. Survive
2. Characteristics
3. Discharge
4. Prenatal, postnatal
5. Breast milk

Part 2

1. Vernix caseosa
2. Caput succedaneum
3. Lanugo

Part 3

1. D
2. F
3. H
4. G
5. A
6. E
7. B
8. C

Part 4

1. T
2. F
3. F
4. F
5. T

Part 5

1. Apgar, weight and length, physical examination
2. 1, 5
3. 8, no
4. Retractions of the chest and xiphoid process, opposition movements in upper and lower chest, nasal flaring, expiratory grunts, and tachypnea
5. Heat loss
6. Before the baby leaves the delivery room he or she receives an identification bracelet (two are applied to the baby and one name band to the mother's wrist).

CHAPTER 67

Part 1

1. 3
2. 5
3. 1
4. 2
5. 4

Part 2

1. Ectopic not dystocia
2. Preeclampsia not hydramnios

3. Eclampsia not gestational diabetes
4. True, no correction needed
5. True, no correction needed

Part 3

1. A
2. A
3. I
4. A
5. I

Part 4

1. Cerclage
2. Amniocentesis
3. Placenta previa
4. Abruptio placenta
5. Dystocia

Part 5

1. D
2. E
3. B
4. C
5. A

CHAPTER 68

Part 1

1. Hemolytic conditions, birth injuries
2. Chemically dependent newborn
3. Dependency
4. Birth, resuscitation, nursery
5. Care planning

Part 2

1. Anencephaly—D
2. Epispadias—C
3. Thrush—E
4. Spina bifida—A
5. Hydrocephalus—B

Part 3

1. T
2. F
3. T
4. F
5. T

Part 4

1. A
2. A
3. A
4. I
5. I
6. A

Part 5

1. Large, hypoglycemia.
2. Any three of the following: meconium or amniotic fluid aspiration, cyanosis, physiologic jaundice, hydration, necrotizing enterocolitis, hypoglycemia
3. See sample care plan: frequent monitoring of breath sounds, respiratory rate, skin color, supportive measures, oxygen therapy through plastic hood, and careful suctioning as needed
4. Any two of the following (examples of effects provided, see text for details).
   Alcohol—fetal alcohol syndrome includes growth deficiency, cardiac anomalies, etc.
   Cocaine and crack—newborn withdrawal, small strokes in utero, and possibly SIDS
   Heroin—newborn withdrawal
   Marijuana—short gestation, precipitate labor, and a higher incidence of meconium staining and aspiration

CHAPTER 69

Part 1

1. 3
2. 1
3. 4
4. 2

Part 2

1. Mind, spirit, core
2. Diagnosing causes, treatment
3. Enjoy, engage

Part 3

1. Contraception
2. Impotence
3. Orgasm
4. Priapism
5. Dyspareunia

Part 4

1. E
2. A
3. B
4. C
5. F
6. D

Part 5

1. I
2. I
3. A
4. A
5. A

Part 6

1. Appetite, excitement, orgasm
2. Lifestyle, effectiveness, or risk
3. Any three of the following: Norplant is an implant that can protect against pregnancy for up to 5 years; Depo-provera injections given every 3 months will prevent ovulation; oral contraceptives prevent ovulation; the morning after pill prevents implantation of the fertilized egg.
4. Intrauterine, barrier, sterilization

CHAPTER 70

Part 1

1. 1
2. 4
3. 6
4. 2
5. 3
6. 5

Part 2

1. Age-related, family, preparation
2. Play
3. Milestones, delays
4. Young

Part 3

1. Pediatrics
2. Immunization
3. Pediatrician

Part 4

1. D
2. A
3. E
4. B
5. C

Part 5

1. Restraints, 1, 2, every
2. NEVER
3. Protect
4. a. Hep B-1—birth to 2 months
   b. Polio—2 months, 4 months, 12 to 18 months, and 4 to 6 years
   c. Hib—2 months, 4 months, 6 months, 12 to 15 months
   d. Measles, mumps, rubella—12 to 15 months, 4 to 6 years, or 11 to 12 years
   e. Diphtheria, tetanus, pertussis—2 months, 4

months, 6 months, 15 to 18 months, 4 to 6 years, Td—11 to 12, 14 to 16 years
5. Any four of the following: restlessness, panic, tachycardia, tachypnea, nasal flaring, wheezing, stridor, change in color, expiratory grunt, retractions, gasping and shallow, labored breaths, head bobbing

Part 6

1. C
2. B
3. D
4. A

CHAPTER 71

Part 1

1. Trauma
2. Eyes
3. Neurologic
4. Skin
5. Cardiovascular
6. Metabolic, nutritional
7. Immunization
8. Lack, supervision
9. Fluid, electrolyte, dehydration
10. Meningomyelocele

Part 2

1. T
2. F
3. T
4. F
5. F

Part 3

1. Encephalocele
2. Marasmus
3. Celiac disease
4. Reye's syndrome

Part 4

1. D
2. A
3. E
4. F
5. C
6. B

Part 5

1. I
2. A
3. A
4. I
5. A
6. I
7. I
8. A

Part 6

ventricular septal defect

hypertrophy of right ventricle

stenosis of pulmonary artery

aorta overriding both ventricles

Part 7

1. D
2. C

CHAPTER 72

Part 1

1. Communicable
2. Reproductive, system
3. Gastrointestinal
4. Skin
5. Musculoskeletal
6. Endocrine
7. Anorexia, bulimia
8. Acne, menstrual, emotional

Part 2

1. Retinitis pigmentosa
2. Cataplexy
3. Somnambulism
4. Mittelschmerz
5. Hypersomnia
6. Impetigo contagiosa

Part 3

1. Narcolepsy
2. Mononucleosis
3. Malocclusion
4. Orthodontia

Part 4

1. E
2. B
3. D
4. C
5. A

Part 5

1. A
2. A
3. I
4. A
5. I
6. A
7. I
8. A

Part 6

1. D
2. C
3. B

CHAPTER 73

Part 1

1. 4
2. 5

3. 2
4. 1
5. 3

Part 2

1. Alcohol, drugs
2. Cerebral palsy, Duchenne muscular dystrophy
3. Self-esteem
4. Expected perfect child

Part 3

1. Autism
2. Suicide
3. Dysfluency
4. Dyslexia

Part 4

1. A
2. I
3. I
4. A
5. A
6. I
7. I
8. A

Part 5

1. A
2. D
3. C
4. E
5. B

Part 6

1. Genetic, acquired
2. Children with Down syndrome have round small short heads, faces with flattened profile, and ears that are small and low-set; children with fragile X syndrome have abnormally large heads, a face with a long, large, protruding jaw, and ears that are large and protruding.
3. Including the family, involving children in care, keeping up with school, and using community resources

CHAPTER 74

Part 1

1. A
2. D
3. C
4. B
5. C

Part 2

1. Diagnostic
2. Folliculitis and carbuncles
3. Skin grafts
4. Contact dermatitis
5. Dermatology
6. Electrical/radiation
7. Skin
8. Angiomas/nonmalignant
9. Parasitic
10. Cancer

Part 3

1. Nonviable or dead
2. Deep dermal
3. Cannot
4. Completely
5. Nitrogen
6. Bacteria
7. Pigskin
8. Shortening
9. Noncontagious
10. Warts

Part 4

1. Partial
2. Tissue/breathing
3. Resuscitative/rehabilitative
4. Smoke inhalation
5. Infection

CHAPTER 75

Part 1

1. True
2. False Daily weights
3. True
4. True
5. True

Part 2

1. 5.5
2. 75
3. 7.4
4. 135
5. 2

Part 3

1. B
2. C
3. C
4. C
5. A

CHAPTER 76

Part 1

1. F
2. H
3. B
4. G
5. E
6. C
7. H
8. A
9. D
10. B
11. E
12. C
13. G
14. A
15. D

Part 2

1. Benign
2. Immobilizes
3. Decreased
4. Skin
5. Traumatic

Part 3

1. Arthroplasty
2. Prosthesis
3. Sequestration
4. Arthritis
5. Tenosynovitis
6. Arthroscopy
7. Osteomyelitis
8. Ankylosis
9. Scleroderma
10. Dislocation

Part 4

1. B
2. C
3. B
4. A
5. D

Part 5

Nursing Alert—Taped to the halo device in case of emergency (see page 1017)

CHAPTER 77

Part 1

1. Nerve disorders
2. Trauma
3. Nursing process
4. Degenerative disorders
5. Inflammatory disorders

6. Trauma
7. Inflammatory disorders
8. Degenerative disorders
9. Nerve disorders
10. Craniocerebral disorders

Part 2

1. Life-threatening
2. Craniocerebral disorders
3. Level of consciousness
4. Nonmalignant
5. Craniotomy

Part 3

1. True
2. False Inside
3. True
4. False Muscle
5. False Spinal cord as well
6. False High blood pressure
7. False Concussion
8. False Invasive
9. False Headache
10. True

Part 4

All symptoms are those characteristic of Guillain-Barré syndrome.

CHAPTER 78

Part 1

1. C
2. B
3. C
4. B
5. D

Part 2

1. Insulin resistance
2. Acromegaly
3. Pheochromocytoma
4. Chvostek's sign
5. Cushing's syndrome

Part 3

1. Polydipsia
2. Hyperglycemia
3. Polyphagia
4. Hypothyroidism
5. Hypophysectomy
6. Hyperparathyroidism
7. Polyuria

Part 4

Number 4

Part 5

1. Classification
2. Medical treatment
3. Complications
4. Signs and symptoms
5. Client teaching
6. Classification
7. Client teaching
8. Medical treatments
9. Signs and symptoms
10. Complications

CHAPTER 79

Part 1

1. Retina
2. Surgery
3. Outpatient
4. Infectious
5. Environmental

Part 2

1. C
2. B
3. A
4. C
5. B

Part 3

C. Narrow-angle glaucoma

CHAPTER 80

Part 1

1. Blood vessel disorders
2. Common medical treatments
3. Common surgical treatments
4. Heart disorders
5. Blood vessel disorders

Part 2

1. Affected
2. Temporary
3. Some
4. Can
5. Necrosis

Part 3

1. Valve, hemorrhage
2. Dizziness, 6, electrical
3. 15
4. Nonaffected
5. Shellfish, iodine

Part 4

1. D
2. E
3. F

4. A
5. G
6. C
7. B

3. A
4. C
5. A
6. D
7. B
8. E

CHAPTER 81

Part 1

1. True
2. False Red blood cell disorders (anemias)
3. False Lymphatic system
4. True
5. False White blood cell disorders

Part 2

1. Autologous
2. Hemophilia
3. Leukopenia
4. Allogeneic
5. Leukemia

Part 3

1. C
2. B
3. B
4. A
5. D

Part 4

Sickle cell, genetic

CHAPTER 82

Part 1

1. C
2. E

Part 2

1. 7
2. Cured, early
3. Lung
4. Body system
5. four, Sarcoma, lymphoma

Part 3

1. Uncontrolled
2. Not (curative)
3. Decreased
4. Prevent
5. Not (confined)
6. Reduction
7. Primary
8. Cells
9. Cause
10. Connective

Part 4

1. True
2. False When *not* correctly managed *can be*
3. True
4. False Early detection promises the highest rate of survival.
5. True

CHAPTER 83

Part 1

1. Allergic
2. Autoimmune
3. Antigens
4. Antibody
5. T lymphocyte and B cells

Part 2

1. Allergy, allergens
2. 20, severe

Part 3

1. Antigen
2. Immunotherapy
3. Autoimmunity
4. Immunogens
5. Anaphylaxis

Part 4

1. B
2. C
3. B
4. A

CHAPTER 84

Part 1

1. False Usually
2. False (Are) *not*
3. True
4. True

Part 2

1. Retrovirus
2. *Pneumocystis carinii* pneumonia
3. B cells
4. Pandemic
5. Thymus

CHAPTER 85

Part 1

1. D

2. B
3. A
4. D

Part 2

1. Hypoxia
2. Acute rhinitis
3. Irritants, trauma
4. Hay fever
5. Cough, pattern, breath

Part 3

1. H
2. G
3. I
4. B
5. F
6. J
7. A
8. D
9. E
10. C

Part 4

1. False Every 15 minutes
2. True
3. False Number has increased
4. True
5. True

CHAPTER 86

Part 1

1. Supportive
2. Nasal
3. Essential
4. Tracheostomy
5. Medication

Part 2

1. Manual breathing bag

2. Venturi mask
3. Ventilator
4. Partial rebreathing mask
5. Pulse oximeter

Part 3

1. 6 LPM
2. Hyperextend
3. One to one
4. Venturi mask
5. One-third

Part 4

1. 2
2. Adult respiratory distress syndrome (ARDS)

CHAPTER 87

Part 1

1. C
2. D
3. B
4. A
5. B

Part 2

1. Cirrhosis
2. Duodenum
3. Symptomatically
4. Accessory

Part 3

1. C
2. B
3. A
4. B

Part 4

1. True
2. False Are *not*
3. True
4. False Slowly
5. True

CHAPTER 88

Part 1

1. Obstructive
2. Treatable
3. Surgical
4. All
5. Neoplasms

Part 2

1. Cystoscopy
2. Detrusor
3. Cystitis
4. Urologist
5. Dialysis

Part 3

1. D
2. C
3. B
4. B

CHAPTER 89

Part 1

1. Erectile
2. Testicular
3. Structural
4. Torsion
5. 40

Part 2

1. Cryptorchidism
2. Priapism
3. Orchitis
4. Seminoma
5. Hydrocele

Part 3

1. False Detects a glycoprotein
2. True
3. False After puberty
4. True
5. True
6. False 2 weeks
7. False Excluding
8. True
9. False Testicular
10. True

CHAPTER 90

Part 1

1. D
2. E
3. A
4. E
5. B
6. C
7. D
8. A
9. C
10. B

Part 2

1. Metrorrhagia
2. Cystocele
3. Mammoplasty
4. Cervicitis
5. Laparoscopy

Part 3

1. True

2. True
3. False (Amenorrhea)
4. False (More)
5. False (Seldom)

Part 4

1. 40%
2. Chest wall, recurrence

CHAPTER 91

Part 1

1. C
2. E
3. B
4. D
5. B

Part 2

1. Aspiration
2. Caregiver stress
3. Edentulous
4. Friable
5. Presbycusis
6. Respite

Part 3

1. A
2. C
3. B

Part 4

1. Vulnerable adult
2. Elder abuse
3. Any two of the following: person's ability to provide for physical, financial and emotional self-care needs; physical, financial, and emotional support from family and friends; access to healthcare and rehabilitation services; need for protection and supervision

4. Home care, senior day care, retirement complexes, and long-term care facilities
5. Remotivation techniques, recreation, cognitive function, social life and activities, pet therapy, religious support, and use of volunteers

CHAPTER 92

Part 1

1. 1st
2. Types of dementias
3. Palliative
4. Respite

Part 2

1. B
2. H
3. A
4. D
5. C
6. E
7. G
8. F

Part 3

1. A	5. A
2. A	6. A
3. I	7. I
4. I	8. I

Part 4

1. Any three of the following: genetic, viral, toxic, immunologic, trauma, biochemical, or nutritional
2. Short-term, long-term
3. Any two of the following is accurate: cerebral cortex atrophy; loss of neurons; or changes in brain cells
4. Faster, stepwise, conditions
5. Toxic, metabolic
6. Express

CHAPTER 93

Part 1

1. The mental healthcare team
2. Methods of psychiatric therapy
3. Community
4. Major depressive episode
5. Productively

Part 2

1. Affect
2. Akathisia
3. Anhedonia
4. Anxiety
5. Athetoid
6. Catatonia
7. Compulsion
8. Defense mechanism
9. Dual diagnosis
10. Dyskinesia

Part 3

1. Dystonia
2. Functional disorder
3. Milieu therapy
4. Mutism
5. Neuroleptic
6. Perseverate
7. Neuroleptic malignant syndrome (NMS)
8. Oculogyric crisis
9. Psychotropic
10. Schizophrenia

Part 4

1. Depressive
2. Anhedonia
3. Bipolar disorder
4. Any one of the following examples is accurate (see text for greater detail).
   Personality disorder: paranoid, schizoid, schizotypal, antisocial, borderline, histrionic, avoidant, dependent
   Anxiety disorder: panic attacks, phobias, obsessive–compulsive, post-traumatic

Psychosis: schizophrenia, brief psychotic, other substance induced etc, psychosis caused by medical disorder
5. Transportation
6. Remotivation
7. Pet
8. Extrapyramidal
9. Civil, vulnerable, advocacy
10. Physical care, teaching life, occupational

5. Caffeine
6. Physical, genetic, emotional, psychological, mental
7. Denial, rationalization, projection
8. All possible
9. Thiamine (B_1), folic acid (B_9)
10. Physical, cycle

Part 5

1. D
2. A
3. E
4. C
5. B

Part 4

1. D
2. C
3. B

CHAPTER 94

Part 1

1. Substance abuse and chemical dependency
2. Detoxification and recovery
3. Stress, self-esteem
4. Codependent
5. More

CHAPTER 95

Part 1

1. Long-term, independent living
2. Lifestyle option
3. Restrictive
4. Rehabilitation services
5. Rehabilitation

Part 2

1. Agonist therapy
2. Alcohol hallucinosis
3. Aversion therapy
4. Blackouts
5. Chemical dependency
6. Delirium tremens
7. Detoxification
8. Refeeding syndrome
9. Substance abuse
10. Withdrawal

Part 2

1. Assisted living
2. Congregate housing
3. Transdermal electrical nerve stimulation
4. Intermediate care facilities
5. Mainstreaming
6. Neurogenic
7. Orthotics
8. Physiatrist
9. Prosthetics
10. Skilled nursing facility

Part 3

1. Alcohol, prescribed
2. Tolerance
3. Nicotine
4. Anabolic steroids

Part 3

1. A
2. A
3. I
4. A
5. I
6. I

Part 4

1. Skin breakdown
2. 2
3. Hemiplegic, quadriplegic
4. Strengthening, stretching
5. Basic functional, instrumental

CHAPTER 96

Part 1

1. T
2. F
3. T
4. F
5. F

Part 2

1. Cardioversion
2. Care map
3. Comorbidity
4. Disease management program
5. Ports
6. Vertical client

Part 3

1. Assist with
2. Call in
3. Measure
4. Primary
5. Assist with

Part 4

1. A
2. I
3. A
4. I
5. I

Part 5

1. Hospital-based, registries, temporary, hospice
2. Any two of the following: client's home, nursing home, or other facility such as a jail
3. Long-term
4. Furnish services in accordance with agency policies; prepare clinical and progress notes, assist physicians and RNs to perform specialized procedures; prepare equipment and materials for treatments, observing aseptic techniques as required; and assist clients in learning appropriate self-care techniques.
5. See Box 96-2, examples include: wear a name badge, telephone clients in advance, ask client to properly secure menacing pets, keep change for emergency telephone calls, keep vehicles in good working order with plenty of gas.

CHAPTER 97

Part 1

1. Evolution of the hospice movement
2. Hospice concept
3. Role of the hospice nurse
4. Respite
5. Relief, side effects

Part 2

1. Ablative surgery or surgical ablation
2. Adjuvant
3. Bereavement
4. Debulking
5. Hospice
6. Palliative care
7. Primary caregivers
8. Respite
9. Somnolent
10. Titration

Part 3

1. T
2. F
3. F

4. T
5. T
6. F
7. F
8. T
9. T
10. T

Part 4

1. Physical, psychological/emotional, social/cultural, spiritual
2. Alleviate, quality, unpleasant
3. Any three of the criteria in Box 97-1. The following are examples: life expectancy is usually no more than 6 months from date of admission, admission can be directed primarily toward meeting the needs of the family; and in most cases the patient and family have agreed on DNR/DNI status.
4. Left alone, pain
5. Observe, discuss

CHAPTER 98

Part 1

1. E
2. F
3. D
4. D
5. C

Part 2

1. Expanding
2. Right, wrong, effective
3. Nationally

Part 3

1. Autocratic
2. Bureaucratic
3. Career mobility
4. Democratic
5. Laissez-faire
6. Telephone triage

Part 4

1. Therapeutic rehabilitation, preventive
2. Any five of the following: assessment, planning, implementation, evaluation, member of the discipline, political activism
3. Shift, assigning, acuity, emergencies
4. Make rounds
5. All, stat
6. Verbal, telephone

Part 5

1. A
2. I
3. I
4. I
5. A

CHAPTER 99

Part 1

1. Employment
2. Job-seeking skills
3. Search, apply, continuing education
4. Beginning, learning
5. Organizations, communities

Part 2

1. Commencement
2. Interstate endorsement
3. Probationary
4. Reciprocity
5. Registry
6. Resumé
7. Telehealth

Part 3

1. NCLEX
2. Differs

3. Any five of the following (see text for greater detail).

Hospitals: LPN or RN

Extended care facilities: LPN or RN

Public health nursing and home care: RN

Private duty, hospice, chemical dependency and detox nursing, mental health, residential treatment center, prison or jail, physician's office, day-surgery clinics, telehealth, occupational health and industrial nursing, armed forces, schools, pairs nursing, Head Start programs, weight loss clinics, or camp nursing (all could be LPN or RN)

4. Practical nursing programs: LPNs and nonbaccalaureate RNs

Operating Rooms: both LPN or RN

Dialysis nursing, hyperbaric medicine, pharmaceutical sales, insurance companies, veterinary clinics, chiropractic clinics, dental or ophthalmology clinics, emergency rescue, self-employment (both might be employed)

5. Job application and resumé preparation, interview, aptitude, and test taking skills

6. Jobs, newspapers, bulletin boards, nursing journals, Internet

Part 4

1. I
2. A
3. A
4. I
5. A
6. A
7. I
8. A